RENAL DIET AND SMOOTHIE CLEANSER GUIDE

ELEVATE YOUR WELL-BEING - A TRANSFORMATIVE EXPLORATION INTO KIDNEY HEALTH WITH DIETARY WISDOM AND SMOOTHIE BRILLIANCE

Nancy Ware

TABLE OF CONTENT

INTRODUCTION

Chronic Kidney Disease (CKD) is a frightening story in terms of health issues, casting shadows of uncertainty and lifestyle constraints on people who have been diagnosed. However, Kane's amazing story stands as a beacon of hope, demonstrating how a planned approach to food and the use of renal-friendly smoothies played a critical role in rewriting his health narrative.

Kane's journey begins with the stark reality of a CKD diagnosis, a moment that had the potential to define the rest of his life as one of constraint and sacrifice. Faced with the prospect of typical medical interventions and their associated problems, Kane explored an alternate path—one that centered on utilizing nature's power and nutrition to naturally supports his kidneys.

The foundation of Kane's transformative journey is his dedication to comprehending the complexities of a renal diet. With an understanding of the effects of salt, potassium, and phosphorus on kidney function, Kane modified his food choices to reduce the strain on his kidneys. His dietary strategy included not only avoiding high-sodium and processed meals but also emphasizing the consumption of nutrient-dense foods such as high-quality proteins, and low-phosphorus fruits and vegetables.

However, what distinguished Kane's approach was his incorporation of renal-friendly smoothies into his daily regimen. Recognizing the potential of these nutrient-dense mixtures to augment his diet, Kane experimented with numerous combinations that not only met his precise nutritional requirements but also added a burst of taste to his culinary range. Low-potassium and low-phosphorus components became the focus of his smoothie creations, demonstrating that a particular taste does not have to be sacrificed for the goal of renal health.

The guide Kane followed didn't stop at recipes; it extended to incorporating smoothies strategically throughout his day. From stimulating breakfast blends to fulfilling snack options, Kane learned that these smoothies were more than simply a healthy supplement; they became an integrated and pleasurable part of his routine.

Kane's path highlights the significant link between lifestyle choices and renal health. His dedication to regular exercise, attentive hydration, and stress management emphasizes the comprehensive character of his approach. It's more than just following a diet; it's about living a holistic lifestyle that nurtures the body and supports kidney function.

This story is not unique to Kane; it serves as a guide for anybody dealing with the hardships of chronic kidney disease. It reveals the possibility of a transformative journey—one that surpasses the constraints commonly linked with chronic health disorders. Kane's tale acts as an inspiration, urging people to seek natural, holistic solutions in their search for better kidney health. Via this book, we will go on a journey of understanding, empowerment, and realization that a shift in the health narrative is possible via educated choices, resilience, and the nourishing power of nature's richness.

CHAPTER ONE

Brief overview of renal health

Renal health, also known as kidney health, is an important aspect of general well-being, as it helps to maintain internal balance, regulate blood pressure, and eliminate waste from the body. Understanding the fundamentals of renal health is critical for anyone looking to protect and improve the function of their kidneys.

The kidneys are two bean-shaped organs positioned on either side of the spine in the lower back. They are crucial to the urinary system and perform a variety of vital tasks. The kidneys' principal function is to filter the blood, eliminating waste materials and excess fluids to produce urine. This process aids in the maintenance of an appropriate electrolyte balance, such as sodium and potassium, as well as the regulation of fluid levels in the body.

The glomerular filtration rate (GFR) is an important indicator of renal health since it measures how well the kidneys filter waste from the blood. A healthy GFR ensures that the kidneys function efficiently. Chronic Kidney Disease (CKD) develops when the kidneys are damaged or unable to filter blood adequately for an extended period. Monitoring and maintaining a healthy GFR is critical to preventing the advancement of kidney-related problems.

The complicated network of microscopic blood arteries called nephrons within the kidneys aids in the filtering process. Nephrons filter the blood, reabsorbing important chemicals such as water and electrolytes, and excreting the residual waste as urine. Any interruption in this delicate equilibrium might lead to problems and jeopardize kidney function.

A variety of factors can have an impact on renal health, and understanding these elements is critical for preventive care. Lifestyle factors such as nutrition, exercise, and hydration have a substantial impact on kidney function. High sodium, phosphorus, and potassium diets can put a strain on the kidneys, particularly in people with pre-existing problems. Regular physical activity improves cardiovascular health and lowers the risk of diseases that can lead to kidney difficulties.

Systemic diseases like diabetes and hypertension can have a significant impact on renal function. These disorders can harm blood vessels and nephrons, speeding up the progression of kidney disease. Regular health screenings, such as blood pressure monitoring and renal function tests, are critical for early detection and treatment of any problems.

The anatomy of the kidneys

Bean-Shaped Maestros

Kidneys, which resemble beans, are paired organs located on either side of the spine. Despite their unassuming look, they perform a variety of tasks that contribute to the overall harmony of body systems.

Nephrones

The kidneys include an ensemble of microscopic dancers known as nephrons. These small structures filter blood meticulously, providing a harmonious balance of electrolytes and hydration levels.

Glorious Glomerulus.

Consider the glomerulus to be the stage spotlight for the nephron. It is a network of small blood arteries that performs the amazing task of filtering blood, separating important nutrients from waste materials and going for the grand exit.

Tubular Tale.

As filtered blood components exit the glomerulus, they travel through the tubules, reabsorbing water and vital nutrients. Consider it the nephron's method of ensuring that nothing valuable goes to waste.

Ureteric Ushers.

After the filtration extravaganza, the ushering begins. The ureters, like devoted ushers, direct the refined pee to its final destination: the bladder.

Renal artery

The renal artery supplies oxygenated blood to the kidneys, powering their vital functions and supporting the delicate filtration processes required for overall health.

Renal Cortex

The renal cortex, the kidney's outer layer, contains critical structures such as glomeruli and convoluted tubules, which play an important role in blood filtration and urine production.

Renal Medulla

The renal medulla, located within the kidney, contains renal pyramids that help to concentrate urine and regulate water and electrolyte balance.

Renal papilla

The renal papilla is the peak of the renal pyramid, when urine from the collecting ducts enters the renal pelvis, beginning its journey to the ureter.

Renal Pelvis

The renal pelvis serves as a storage for urine, collecting filtered fluid from the renal papillae and delivering it to the bladder via the ureter.

Renal Vein

The renal vein transports deoxygenated blood, which contains filtered waste and excess fluid, away from the kidneys and returns it to the circulatory system for purification.

A Fun Approach to Renal Health

Hydration Tango.

Consider a vibrant tango between kidneys and water levels. Proper fluid intake helps to eliminate waste and maintain the delicate electrolyte balance, ensuring a smooth dance experience.

Blood Pressure Ballet.

Kidneys are beautiful performers in the blood pressure ballet. They control blood pressure by altering fluid levels and releasing a small amount of renin. What was the result? A consistent performance of cardiovascular health.

Electrolyte Circus.

Imagine the nephron's tubular parts as a lively circus. Electrolytes (sodium, potassium, and others) perform daring feats of balance, keeping the body's internal circus vibrant and well-coordinated.

PH Jamboree

The kidneys throw a pH party to keep the body's acid-base balance in check. This guarantees that our internal environment remains stable, preventing any uncontrollable alterations in the body's chemical balance.

Detox Waltz.

The kidneys do a cleansing waltz, tirelessly eliminating the body of waste materials and pollutants. It's their method of keeping the body's internal dance floor clean and ready for the next performance.

Importance of a renal diet and smoothie cleanser

The kidneys, those inconspicuous but critical organs, perform an important role in maintaining internal balance. An intentional and careful approach to supporting these bean-shaped wonders with a renal diet and smoothie cleanser is essential for maintaining good renal health.

The Importance of a Renal Diet:

1. Managing Sodium, Potassium, and Phosphorus

A renal diet is carefully designed to control salt, potassium, and phosphorus intake. By managing these nutrients, the diet reduces the load on the kidneys, preventing problems and the evolution of illnesses such as Chronic Kidney Disease.

2. Maintaining protein balance

High-quality proteins are carefully integrated to maintain a precise equilibrium. This not only promotes overall health but also minimizes the accumulation of waste products, which can strain damaged kidneys.

3. Fluid Intake Regulation

A renal diet contains fluid intake guidelines to keep the kidneys from working too hard. Proper hydration is essential, maintaining a balance between getting enough fluids for health and avoiding undue stress on renal function.

4. Supporting Blood Pressure Management

Hypertension is both the cause and the result of renal problems. A renal diet helps to manage blood pressure, lower the risk of kidney impairment, and promote cardiovascular health.

5. Reducing Phosphorus Load

Foods high in phosphorus are restricted to reduce the risk of problems. This is especially important because increased phosphorus levels can lead to bone and heart problems in people with impaired kidney function.

The Function of a Smoothie Cleanser

1. Nutrient-dense Hydration

Smoothies, when properly prepared, are a refreshing and nutrient-dense source of water. This is especially advantageous for people with kidney disease, who may need to limit their fluid consumption.

2. Incorporating Renal-Friendly Ingredients

Renal-friendly smoothies prioritize components that are low in potassium and phosphorus. This ensures a delicious and pleasurable addition to the diet while maintaining kidney health.

3. Managing Appetite and Nutrition.

Smoothies are a practical and delicious option for persons with limited appetites to increase nutritional consumption. This is critical for maintaining energy levels and improving overall health.

4. Variety in Nutrient Intake

Smoothie cleansers provide a varied dose of important nutrients, vitamins, and minerals. This variant meets the body's general nutritional demands while also responding to the unique needs of renal health.

5. An Appealing Approach to Dietary Compliance

Renal diets can sometimes be seen as restrictive. Smoothies, on the other hand, provide a tasty and innovative way to follow dietary rules, making the overall approach to renal health more fun.

The benefits of a renal diet and smoothie cleanser cannot be emphasized in terms of kidney health. These dietary methods are more than just limits; they are strategic tools that enable people to actively engage in the preservation and improvement of their kidney health. Individuals who embrace these activities start on a journey that nourishes their nephrons, promotes general health, and produces a deep sense of well-being.

Why kidney health matters

Kidney health is a matter of profound significance, as these remarkable organs play a crucial role in maintaining the overall balance and well-being of the body. The kidneys are more than just filters; they are complicated regulators that influence a variety of physiological processes, thus their health is critical to systemic balance.

1. Filtration and Waste Elimination

The filtration of blood is crucial to kidney function, as it ensures the elimination of waste materials and excess fluids. This detoxification function is critical for preventing the accumulation of toxic compounds that could endanger the body's internal environment.

2. Electrolyte and Fluid Balance.

The kidneys are adept at controlling electrolytes such as salt and potassium, which are essential for maintaining adequate fluid balance. Their capacity to fine-tune these concentrations prevents dehydration or the retention of extra fluids, which helps to keep blood pressure constant.

3. Blood Pressure Regulation

Renin, a kidney hormone, is essential for blood pressure regulation. Healthy kidney function is critical for maintaining this delicate balance, avoiding hypertension, and lowering the risk of cardiovascular disease.

4. Red Blood Cell Production.

The kidneys generate erythropoietin, a hormone that promotes the formation of red blood cells. This ensures that tissues and organs receive appropriate oxygen, which promotes general vitality.

5. Metabolic Waste Removal

Aside from filtering blood, the kidneys remove metabolic wastes, including acids, that might build during cellular processes. This helps to maintain the body's acid-base balance.

6. Prevent Chronic Kidney Disease (CKD)

Kidney health is critical for preventing the beginning and progression of Chronic Kidney Disease. Individuals who follow lifestyle measures that promote renal well-being can dramatically minimize their risk of having this devastating ailment.

7. Impact on the Urinary System

The kidneys are essential to the urinary system, generating urine and maintaining adequate excretion. Kidney stones and urinary tract infections highlight the necessity of maintaining proper kidney function.

8. Overall health and longevity.

Healthy kidneys promote general health and lifespan. Their involvement in maintaining internal balance and supporting critical biological functions emphasizes their importance to an individual's overall well-being.

Common Kidney Health Concerns.

1. Chronic kidney disease (CKD).

CKD is a degenerative condition in which the kidneys gradually lose their function over time. It is commonly connected with conditions such as diabetes and hypertension, demanding careful management to prevent further deterioration.

2. Kidney stones.

These are hard deposits that form in the kidneys and can cause considerable pain while passing through the urinary tract. Dehydration, nutritional factors, and genetics all contribute to their growth.

3. Urinary tract infection (UTI).

Urinary tract infections can result in kidney issues. Prompt treatment is necessary to keep infection from spreading to these vital organs.

Maintaining Kidney Health

1. Stay Hydrated.

Proper hydration promotes healthy kidney function. It promotes efficient waste removal and reduces the risk of kidney stones.

2. Follow a healthy diet.

A well-balanced diet rich in fruits, vegetables, and lean proteins yet low in sodium and processed foods improves kidney function. Following a renal diet, if necessary, can be beneficial.

3. Regular exercise.

Physical activity boosts cardiovascular health and reduces the incidence of kidney-related disorders.

4. Regular Checkups

Periodic health checks, such as blood pressure monitoring and renal function tests, help to detect and address problems as early as possible.

Kidney health is crucial to overall well-being. Understanding kidney function, being aware of frequent concerns, and maintaining a healthy lifestyle all contribute to the preservation of these vital organs. Regular checkups and aggressive management are essential for keeping a healthy and resilient renal system.

Connection between lifestyle and renal health

The complex relationship between lifestyle choices and renal health emphasizes the importance of everyday activities on kidney function and well-being. The kidneys, which filter blood, regulate fluid balance, and eliminate waste, are heavily influenced by lifestyle factors such as food, physical activity, hydration, stress management, and other health-related decisions.

Diet and Nutrition

Dietary choices are an important aspect of renal health because they support normal kidney function. An individual's daily dietary intake has a substantial impact on the kidneys' capacity to perform their complicated functions. High salt, phosphorus, and potassium levels in the diet might strain the kidneys and cause difficulties. A renal-friendly diet, which is frequently recommended for people with kidney problems, promotes the consumption of high-quality proteins, restricts processed foods, and takes into account individual health demands. This personalized approach not only improves kidney function but also addresses the specific dietary requirements of patients with poor renal health.

Hydration.

Adequate hydration is necessary for the kidneys to operate properly. Drinking adequate water helps the body eliminate toxins and waste products more efficiently. Dehydration, on the other hand, can increase the concentration of urine, thereby contributing to the production of kidney stones. Consistent and enough water intake provides appropriate filtration, aids in the prevention of urinary tract infections, and promotes overall kidney function.

Physical Activity.

Regular physical exercise is not only good for your heart, but it also helps your kidneys function properly. Exercise supports good blood pressure and circulation, lowering the risk of kidney-related illnesses. Increased blood flow during physical exercise promotes efficient filtration mechanisms, which contribute to the preservation of good renal function.

Maintaining a Healthy Weight.

Obesity poses a considerable risk for renal disease. Excess body weight can increase the risk of diabetes and hypertension, both of which can affect kidney function over time. Adopting a balanced diet and regular exercise helps with weight management and prevents kidney-related issues.

Blood Pressure Management

Hypertension is the major cause of renal disease. Lifestyle changes, such as eating a low-sodium diet, exercising regularly, and practicing stress-reduction techniques, can help manage blood pressure and maintain kidney health. These actions not only help to prevent renal disease, but they also have a larger impact on cardiovascular health.

Stress Management.

Chronic stress has been associated with the development and progression of renal disease. Stress management strategies such as meditation, yoga, and mindfulness practices are not only good for your mental health, but they also improve renal health. These activities can lessen the physiological consequences of stress on the body, creating a balanced environment for good kidney function.

Avoid smoking and excessive alcohol consumption.

Smoking and excessive alcohol intake are known to cause kidney impairment. Quitting smoking and limiting alcohol consumption are critical steps toward improving overall health, including renal function. These lifestyle adjustments can reduce the risk of kidney-related diseases caused by these unhealthy habits.

Regular Health Check-Ups

Routine health examinations aid in the early diagnosis of probable renal problems. Monitoring blood pressure, renal function tests, and other pertinent measurements enables rapid intervention. Early identification allows healthcare practitioners to take the required steps to prevent the progression of kidney disease and preserve renal function.

Medication Adherence.

Adherence to prescribed drugs is critical for persons managing illnesses such as diabetes or hypertension, as it affects both overall health and kidney function. Proper management of these disorders through medication and lifestyle changes is an important part of sustaining kidney health.

The complicated association between lifestyle choices and renal health emphasizes the significance of taking a comprehensive approach to well-being. Recognizing the influence of daily choices on kidney function allows people to make proactive efforts to protect these essential organs. A kidney-friendly lifestyle, which includes a well-balanced diet, regular exercise, hydration, stress management, and other health-promoting activities, not only promotes normal renal function but also overall vitality and longevity. Individuals who understand and embrace these ideas can live a resilient and active life while protecting the health of their kidneys.

CHAPTER TWO

RENAL DIET GUIDE

Understanding the Renal Diet

Understanding the renal diet is critical for anyone dealing with kidney health issues. This customized diet is designed to manage illnesses such as Chronic renal Disease (CKD) by prioritizing careful control of particular nutrients to reduce renal stress. To maintain fluid balance, sodium consumption is limited, and high-potassium foods such as bananas and oranges are consumed in moderation to avoid electrolyte imbalance. To avoid difficulties, the renal diet focuses on high-quality protein sources such as lean meats and eggs while reducing phosphorus-rich meals. Portion control and fluid intake tracking are essential components in promoting a balanced nutritional approach.

Educating oneself about the subtleties of the renal diet enables people to make informed dietary decisions, ensuring that meals meet their specific health demands. Consultation with healthcare professionals, such as dietitians or nephrologists, is essential for tailored advice and changes. Individuals who understand and follow the principles of the renal diet not only manage their kidney health but also promote general well-being by making informed decisions that support optimal renal function and quality of life.

Overview of renal dietary restrictions

A thorough grasp of renal dietary restrictions is essential for people managing kidney health issues, especially those with Chronic Kidney Disease (CKD). Renal dietary limitations aim to reduce renal stress by carefully controlling the consumption of key nutrients. This comprehensive strategy seeks to protect kidney function while also improving overall well-being. Let's get into the finer points of these restrictions:

Sodium Restriction

Sodium restriction is essential in the renal diet since it has a direct impact on blood pressure and fluid balance. High sodium intake might cause hypertension, perhaps worsening kidney problems. To avoid putting too much strain on the kidneys, processed foods, canned items, and high-sodium condiments are limited. This restriction is a critical preventive approach for treating hypertension and reducing fluid retention.

Potassium moderation

Potassium, an essential electrolyte, should be consumed in moderation in the renal diet. High-potassium foods like bananas, oranges, and potatoes are delicious, but they can cause hyperkalemia, which is when potassium levels rise. This illness can upset the delicate balance of electrolytes, potentially affecting heart function. Limiting potassium intake is critical for maintaining correct electrolyte balance and avoiding problems.

Phosphate Management

Excess phosphorus consumption is a problem for those with kidney disease since reduced kidney function might make it difficult to excrete phosphorus effectively. Elevated phosphorus levels can lead to consequences such as bone and cardiovascular disease. To regulate phosphorus levels and avoid potential issues, the renal diet restricts phosphorus-rich foods such as dairy, nuts, seeds, and certain processed foods.

Protein Control.

While protein is essential for overall health, excessive protein consumption can strain the kidneys by producing extra waste products. The renal diet achieves balance by promoting high-quality proteins derived from lean meats, eggs, and seafood. However, protein consumption is limited to avoid overloading the kidneys with excessive waste. This careful balance ensures that people receive the necessary nutrients without jeopardizing renal function.

Fluid Regulation.

Controlling fluid intake is frequently stressed, especially in the advanced stages of CKD. For people with impaired kidney function, controlling fluid intake helps to reduce fluid retention and consequences including oedema. Fluid control is an important element of the renal diet, and individuals must be cautious of their daily liquid intake.

Portion Control.

Proper portion control is an essential component of the renal diet. It goes beyond limiting individual foods to regulating overall calorie intake. Controlling portion sizes helps to reduce the accumulation of waste products from digestion, which supports kidney function while maintaining a balanced nutritional profile.

Nutrient-dense options

Despite constraints, the renal diet promotes nutrient-dense foods. Fruits, vegetables, and whole grains are valued for their vitamins and minerals. These nutrient-dense alternatives supply critical nutrients without exceeding dietary limits. The emphasis is on maximizing nutrition within the set parameters to promote overall health.

Individualized Plans

Renal dietary limits are not standard; they are tailored to an individual's specific health conditions, stage of kidney disease, and nutritional requirements. Consulting with a healthcare expert or qualified dietitian is essential for adjusting the diet to individual needs. A tailored plan ensures that dietary limitations are consistent with the person's overall health goals and lifestyle.

Regular monitoring and adjustments.

The dynamic nature of kidney health needs continuous monitoring and modifications to the renal diet. Regular health checks, blood tests, and kidney function assessments provide information about the food plan's success. Based on these findings, healthcare providers can make informed decisions to meet evolving health demands and avoid consequences.

Educational Support.

Educational support is an important part of navigating renal dietary restrictions. Individuals receive materials, training, and continuing guidance to help them understand and follow dietary recommendations. Individuals who are empowered with knowledge about their nutritional needs are better equipped to make informed decisions, participate actively in their health management, and improve their quality of life.

The complete discussion of renal dietary limitations emphasizes the delicate balance required for efficient kidney health management. These constraints are not simply limitations, but rather purposeful strategies designed to preserve renal function, reduce problems, and promote general well-being. Individuals who understand and adhere to the principles of the renal diet actively participate in their health journey, making educated decisions that support optimal renal function and improve their overall quality of life.

Importance of managing sodium, potassium, and phosphorus intake

The significance of controlling sodium, potassium, and phosphorus consumption cannot be emphasized, especially for people with kidney-related disorders such as Chronic Kidney Disease (CKD). These vital electrolytes play critical roles in overall health, and careful control is essential for maintaining good kidney function and avoiding problems. Let's look at the significance of handling each of these elements:

Sodium Management.

Blood Pressure Control: Sodium, a crucial component of table salt, directly affects blood pressure. High salt intake is connected to hypertension, which is a major cause of kidney injury. Individuals can control their blood pressure and lower their risk of renal problems by limiting their sodium consumption.

Fluid Balance: Sodium regulates the body's fluid balance. Excess sodium can cause fluid retention, which contributes to oedema and increases the stress on the kidneys. Proper salt control promotes a healthy fluid balance and decreases strain on the kidneys.

Oedema Prevention: One of the most prevalent symptoms of renal disease is oedema or swelling caused by fluid retention. Sodium management is essential for minimizing oedema, improving general comfort, and maintaining kidney health.

Potassium Regulation.

Electrolyte Balance: Potassium is a critical electrolyte for many physiological functions, including muscular contractions and nerve impulses. However, too much potassium can disturb electrolyte balance, causing irregular cardiac rhythms. Proper control ensures that the electrolytes operate optimally.

Heart Health: Elevated potassium levels can harm the heart, potentially leading to arrhythmias. Managing potassium intake is critical for preventing cardiac problems and maintaining cardiovascular health, particularly for people with impaired kidney function.

Hyperkalemia, or increased potassium levels, offers serious health hazards. Individuals can avoid developing this illness by carefully controlling their potassium consumption, which can have major effects on kidney health and overall well-being.

Phosphorus Control

While phosphorus is necessary for bone health, excessive amounts can cause complications in those with kidney disease. Elevated phosphorus levels can lead to bone and cardiovascular problems. Managing phosphorus consumption is crucial for maintaining bone health and avoiding issues.

Calcium-Phosphorus Balance: An imbalance in the calcium-phosphorus ratio can disrupt mineral metabolism, potentially resulting in calcification of blood vessels and soft tissues. Proper phosphorus management helps to maintain this delicate balance, which benefits overall vascular health.

Prevention of Secondary Hyperparathyroidism: High phosphorus levels can cause secondary hyperparathyroidism, a disorder in which the parathyroid glands become overactive. This can have a domino impact on bone health and kidney function, making phosphorus management essential.

Overall Significance

Kidney Function Preservation: Managing sodium, potassium, and phosphorus all help to keep the kidneys working. Uncontrolled levels of these electrolytes can cause kidney injury, hence their regulation is an important part of kidney health management.

Complication Prevention: Proper sodium, potassium, and phosphorus intake help to avoid complications linked with renal illness, such as hypertension, fluid imbalances, electrolyte abnormalities, and bone difficulties.

Individuals can enjoy a higher quality of life if they actively manage their electrolytes. Proper regulation promotes general health, lowers the likelihood of symptoms and consequences, and improves well-being.

Strategies for Management

Dietary Modification: Following a renal-friendly diet entails carefully selecting foods to limit salt, potassium, and phosphorus intake. This could include reducing processed foods, choosing low-sodium options, and being cautious of high-potassium or high-phosphorus foods.

Fluid Management: Keeping track of your fluid intake is critical for maintaining sodium and fluid balance. Adequate hydration prevents dehydration and promotes normal kidney function.

Individuals with kidney issues should engage closely with healthcare specialists, such as dietitians and nephrologists, to receive tailored advice and make dietary changes based on regular monitoring.

Managing salt, potassium, and phosphorus consumption is essential for kidney health. These electrolytes influence a variety of physiological processes, and careful control is critical for avoiding problems, maintaining renal function, and improving general well-being. Individuals can actively control their kidney health and improve their quality of life by adopting conscious dietary behaviors, staying hydrated, and obtaining medical advice.

Recommended fluid intake

Recommended fluid consumption is an important feature of general health, particularly for kidney function. Adequate hydration is required for many physiological processes, and maintaining an adequate fluid balance is critical for the kidneys' healthy function. Here's a complete summary of suggested fluid intake.

Importance of Hydration

1. Kidney Function.

Adequate hydration is essential for proper kidney function. The kidneys remove waste products and excess fluids from the circulation, resulting in urine. Insufficient fluid consumption can result in concentrated urine, which may contribute to kidney stones and urinary tract infections.

2. Electrolyte Balance.

Hydration is essential for keeping electrolytes balanced. Proper fluid levels help to maintain the equilibrium of vital electrolytes such as sodium and potassium, which are required for many physiological functions, including nerve transmission and muscle contraction.

3. Temperature Regulation.

Hydration is crucial for maintaining body temperature. Sweating is the body's natural cooling function, and regular fluid intake helps prevent dehydration, especially in hot or humid weather.

4. Cognitive Function.

Dehydration can have a severe impact on cognitive function, making it harder to concentrate, alert, and perform well overall. Staying hydrated promotes good brain function.

5. Joint Lubrication.

Fluids help lubricate joints. Proper hydration helps preserve joint health, lowering the risk of stiffness and discomfort.

Determining Recommended Fluid Intake

1. Individual Factors.

Individuals' recommended fluid intake varies depending on age, gender, weight, physical activity level, and overall health. Women who are pregnant or breastfeeding, as well as others living in hot areas, may need to drink more fluids.

2. Climate and Activity Levels

Hot and humid weather, as well as physical exercise, raises the body's hydration requirements. Individuals participating in strenuous exercise should restore fluids lost through sweating to stay hydrated.

3. Medical conditions.

Certain medical disorders, such as kidney stones or urinary tract infections, may require higher fluid consumption as part of the treatment plan. Individuals with cardiac issues or oedema may need to closely watch their fluid intake.

Recommended fluid intake guidelines

1. General Guidelines.

The **"8x8 rule,"** which recommends eight 8-ounce glasses of water per day, is a popular recommendation. Individual demands, however, can differ, and a more tailored approach is frequently advantageous.

2. Adequate Hydration Indicators.

Monitoring urine color can help determine hydration. Clear or light-coloured urine often indicates appropriate hydration, however black urine may indicate dehydration.

3. Thirst response.

Paying attention to your body's thirst cues is critical. Thirst is a natural mechanism that indicates the need for fluid intake, and responding to it aids in maintaining optimum hydration.

4. Hydration from Food

Hydration is not limited to beverages; many meals, particularly fruits and vegetables high in water content, contribute to overall fluid intake.

5. Special considerations

Individuals with certain health issues, such as kidney disease, diabetes, or heart disease, should follow the fluid intake recommendations made by their healthcare provider.

Tips for Staying Hydrated

1. Carry a water bottle.

Keeping a water bottle handy supports continuous hydration throughout the day.

2. Set reminders.

Setting reminders, particularly in a hectic schedule, might encourage regular hydration intake.

3. Include Hydrating Foods.

Incorporating foods with high water content, such as fruits and vegetables, helps with general hydration.

4. Tailor to Individual Needs

Recognizing and regulating fluid intake depending on individual needs, activity levels, and environmental conditions is critical for remaining hydrated.

Recommended fluid intake is a dynamic part of health management that affects a variety of bodily functions.

While generic guidelines exist, personalized approaches that take into account aspects such as age, health issues, and exercise levels are crucial. Regular hydration is not only essential for renal function, but it also benefits general health by promoting cognitive function, joint health, and temperature management. Staying tuned in to your body's signals and implementing tailored measures for maintaining optimal hydration are essential components of a proactive approach to health.

Foods to Include in a Renal Diet

Navigating a renal diet requires careful consideration of which foods to include, which is critical for sustaining kidney health. This specific dietary approach stresses nutrient-dense foods while carefully controlling salt, potassium, and phosphorus intake. A diverse diet rich in fruits, vegetables, lean proteins, and whole grains serves as a basis for maintaining healthy kidney function. Understanding the proper balance promotes a well-rounded and healthy renal diet, which is critical for people living with illnesses such as Chronic Kidney Disease.

High-quality protein sources are vital for a well-balanced and healthy diet because they help maintain muscular health, boost immunological function, and provide essential amino acids. Individuals on a renal diet or those managing diseases such as Chronic Kidney Disease (CKD) must carefully select protein sources to lessen the stress on the kidneys. Here's a complete look at high-quality protein sources:

1. Lean meats.

Skinless poultry, including chicken and turkey, are high in lean protein. Removing the skin reduces the saturated fat content.

Fish: Fatty fish such as salmon, trout, and mackerel include not only high-quality protein but also omega-3 fatty acids, which promote cardiovascular health.

Lean Cuts of Red Meat: Choosing lean cuts of beef, hog, or lamb will help you get enough protein without consuming too much-saturated fat.

2. Eggs

Eggs are a versatile and complete protein source that contains all the necessary amino acids. They also contain minerals like choline and B vitamins.

3. Dairy and dairy alternatives.

Low-fat or fat-free dairy Low-fat or fat-free milk, yogurt, and cheese are rich in protein, calcium, and other vital elements.

Plant-Based Alternatives: For those who are lactose intolerant or follow a plant-based diet, fortified plant-based milk alternatives such as almond, soy, or pea protein milk should be investigated.

4. Legumes: Beans and lentils, including kidney, black, and chickpeas, are high in protein, fiber, vitamins, and minerals.

Soy-based products such as tofu and tempeh are complete protein sources, making them excellent vegetarian and vegan options.

5. Nuts and seeds.

Nuts, such as almonds, walnuts, and pistachios, are a healthful snack since they include both protein and healthy fats.

Chia seeds, flaxseeds, and hemp seeds are high in protein and contain omega-3 fatty acids, which promote heart health.

6. Deli Meats (In Moderation)

Lean Deli Meats: When picking deli meats, choose for lean versions such as turkey or chicken and consume them in moderation to increase protein consumption.

7. Greek Yogurt

Greek yogurt is a high-protein food that also contains probiotics, which promote digestive health.

8. Seafood: Shellfish. Shrimp, crab, and other shellfish are low in fat and high in protein, making them a nutritious seafood alternative.

9. Poultry alternatives

Plant-based alternatives: Plant-based burgers, sausages, and nuggets prepared with soy, pea protein, or mycoprotein can help vegetarians and vegans acquire enough protein.

10. Quinoa

Quinoa is a complete protein source, consisting of all nine necessary amino acids. It's also high in fiber, vitamins, and minerals.

Considerations for a Renal Diet

Phosphorus level: For people on a renal diet, it's important to evaluate the phosphorus level of protein sources, as too much phosphorus can be bad for kidney health.

Salt Moderation: Selecting protein sources with minimal salt concentration is critical for controlling blood pressure and maintaining renal health.

Portion management: Proper portion management is essential for avoiding excessive protein intake, which can strain the kidneys.

Including high-quality protein sources in your diet is critical for general health and well-being. Individuals with unique dietary issues, such as those managing kidney illness, should consult with healthcare practitioners or trained dietitians to customize protein selections to their specific needs. A broad and balanced approach to protein intake promotes adequate nutrition while taking into account the particular needs of each person's health journey.

Individuals with kidney-related problems, particularly those managing illnesses such as Chronic Kidney Disease (CKD), should follow a low-phosphorus diet. Fruits and vegetables are crucial components of this diet, supplying vitamins, minerals, and fiber while limiting phosphorus intake. Here's a complete look at low-phosphorus fruits and vegetables:

Low-Phosphorus Fruit:

1. Apples

Apples are low in phosphorus but strong in fiber and antioxidants, which promote digestive health and overall well-being.

2. Berries (Strawberries, Blueberries, Raspberries)

Berries are high in vitamins, antioxidants, and fiber, making them ideal low-phosphorus foods for people with kidney problems.

3. Pineapple

Pineapple is a low-phosphorus tropical fruit that adds a pleasant and naturally sweet flavor to your diet.

4) Watermelon

Watermelon contains a high water content and is low in phosphorus, making it a hydrating and kidney-friendly fruit.

5. Peach

Peaches are a sweet and delectable fruit that is relatively low in phosphorus, making them an excellent complement to a low-phosphorus diet.

6. Grapes

Grapes are not only low in phosphorus, but they also contain antioxidants that promote heart health.

7. Cranberries

Cranberries, whether fresh or juiced, can be incorporated into a low-phosphorus diet and provide extra benefits to urinary health.

8. plums

Plums are a low-phosphorus stone fruit that can be eaten fresh or dried as prunes. They include fiber and natural sweetness.

Low-Phosphorous Vegetables:

1. Bell Pepper

Bell peppers, whether red, green, or yellow, are low in phosphorus but high in vitamins A and C.

2) Cabbage

Cabbage, including green, red, and Napa types, is a versatile, low-phosphorus vegetable that can be eaten raw or cooked.

3. Cauliflower

Cauliflower is a cruciferous vegetable with minimal phosphorus, making it a healthier alternative to higher-phosphorus choices.

4. Zucchini

Zucchini is a mild-flavored, low-phosphorus vegetable that may be used in a variety of recipes to add texture and nutrition.

5. Radishes

Radishes are crisp, low-phosphorus root vegetables that make a tasty complement to salads or snacks.

6. Kale

Kale is a nutrient-dense leafy green that is low in phosphorus but abundant in vitamins, minerals, and antioxidants.

7. Summer squash

Summer squash cultivars, such as yellow squash, have low phosphorus content and can be used in several cuisines.

8. Eggplants

Eggplant is a low-phosphorus vegetable that may be prepared in numerous ways, delivering a unique and hearty addition to meals.

Considerations for a Low-Phosphorus Diet

1. Portion control

While some fruits and vegetables have lower phosphorus content, portion control is key for managing overall nutritional consumption.

2. Cooking methods

Cooking processes, such as boiling or leaching, can further lower phosphorus levels in certain plants.

3. Variety is Key

Incorporating a variety of low-phosphorus fruits and vegetables ensures a broad nutrient intake, which benefits overall health.

4. Consultation with Dietitian

Individuals with significant dietary limitations, particularly those managing kidney illness, should speak with a qualified dietitian for individualized advice.

Fruits and vegetables with low phosphorus content are essential for a kidney-friendly diet. Individuals can support kidney health while enjoying a tasty and nutrient-rich diet by embracing these options and following a well-balanced and varied nutritional approach. Consult with healthcare specialists or dietitians for individualized advice tailored to your specific health needs.

Whole grains and healthy fats

Whole grains and healthy fats are key components of a balanced and nutritious diet, which promotes general health and well-being. Incorporating these nutrient-dense meals delivers numerous benefits, ranging from heart health to weight management. Let's look at the various features of whole grains and healthy fats in the diet:

Whole grains are nutrient-dense.

Whole grains, such as brown rice, quinoa, oats, and whole wheat, are high in critical elements like fiber, vitamins and minerals. Whole grains are beneficial to general health due to their high nutritional density.

Dietary Fiber

Whole grains are very high in fiber, which is good for your digestion. Fiber helps to maintain regular bowel motions, prevents constipation, and promotes a healthy gut microbiota.

Blood Sugar Regulation

Whole grains have a lower glycemic index than processed grains. This feature helps regulate blood sugar levels, making them an excellent alternative for people with diabetes or those looking to manage their blood sugar.

Heart Health.

Whole grains provide fiber and other elements that promote cardiovascular health. Regular whole grain consumption has been linked to a lower risk of heart disease via improving cholesterol levels and blood pressure.

Weight Management.

The satiating action of fiber in whole grains helps with weight control by increasing a sense of fullness, lowering overall calorie intake, and helping weight loss or maintenance efforts.

Antioxidant Content.

Whole grains include antioxidants, which assist in neutralizing free radicals in the body, protecting against oxidative stress and inflammation.

Bone health

Some whole grains, such as quinoa, include magnesium and other nutrients that promote bone health. Consuming whole grains improves total bone strength.

Versatility

Whole grains are adaptable and may be used in a variety of dishes, from breakfast cereals and salads to side dishes and main courses, giving you plenty of alternatives for a healthy diet.

Healthy fats

Monounsaturated fats.

Monounsaturated fats, which are found in olive oil, avocados, and certain nuts, are heart-healthy fats that have been linked to lower cholesterol and better cardiovascular health.

Polyunsaturated fats.

Fatty fish (salmon, mackerel), flaxseeds, chia seeds, and walnuts are excellent sources of omega-3 and omega-6 fatty acids. These fats are essential for brain health, as they reduce inflammation and promote overall well-being.

Omega 3 Fatty Acids

Fish high in omega-3 fatty acids include salmon and trout. These fats serve an important role in heart health, cognitive function, and the prevention of chronic diseases.

Avocados.

Avocados are high in monounsaturated fats and have a creamy texture. They also contain a variety of vitamins and minerals. They increase satiety and can be a nutritious complement to a variety of cuisines.

Nuts and seeds.

Nuts and seeds including almonds, walnuts, chia seeds, and flaxseeds include healthful fats as well as fiber, protein, and antioxidants.

Coconut oil (in moderation).

Coconut oil, while heavy in saturated fat, can be used in moderation to supplement a healthy diet. It contains medium-chain triglycerides (MCTs), which may provide health advantages.

Plant-based oils.

Olive oil, canola oil, and other plant-based oils contain monounsaturated and polyunsaturated fats. These oils are widely used in cooking and salad dressings.

Nutrient Absorption.

Healthy fats aid in the absorption of fat-soluble vitamins (A, D, E, and K), increasing the body's ability to use these vital nutrients.

Considerations for Inclusion:

1. Moderation.

While healthy fats have several benefits, moderation is essential. Excessive consumption of even good fats can lead to caloric excess and have unforeseen health repercussions.

2. Diverse sources

Consuming a combination of whole grains and healthy fats provides a greater range of nutrients and improves the overall nutritional profile of the diet.

3. Individualized Needs

Dietary requirements vary per individual. Individual health objectives, preferences, and any special health issues should inform the addition of whole grains and healthy fats to the diet.

4. Balanced Diet

Integrating whole grains and healthy fats into a well-balanced diet rich in fruits, vegetables, lean meats, and dairy or dairy alternatives helps to meet overall nutritional requirements.

Incorporating whole grains and healthy fats into your diet is an important part of promoting overall health. These nutrient-dense foods support a variety of biological processes, including cardiovascular health and weight control, as well as important nutrients for bone health and cognitive function. A balanced and diverse approach to nutrition, tailored to individual needs, delivers a well-rounded and healthy diet that promotes long-term well-being.

Foods to Limit or Avoid

Navigating a health-conscious diet entails not just enjoying nutrient-dense foods, but also being aware of which to limit or avoid. Certain diets heavy in sodium, refined carbohydrates, saturated fats, and excessive phosphorus can be detrimental to general health. Individuals managing chronic kidney disease (CKD) must understand and restrict specific food items. Limiting processed meals, sugary beverages, and red meat consumption while controlling salt and phosphorus intake benefits kidney function. This introduction lays the groundwork for a thorough examination of foods to limit or avoid, allowing people to make informed dietary decisions for maximum health and the management of specific health conditions.

High-sodium foods

High-sodium meals are a major health concern, especially since high sodium consumption has been related to a variety of health conditions such as hypertension, heart disease, and renal problems. Although sodium is an essential mineral, modern diets frequently include far too much of it. Understanding and identifying high-sodium foods is critical for those who want to control their blood pressure, improve their heart health, and reduce their risk of renal disease. Here's a detailed look at high-sodium foods:

1. Processed and packaged foods.

Canned soups and broths are frequently laden with sodium for flavor improvement and preservation.

Frozen Meals: To maintain flavor and shelf life, many frozen dinners and snacks include high salt levels.

2. condiments and sauces

Soy sauce, which is widely used in a variety of cuisines, contains extraordinarily high levels of sodium.

Ketchup and barbecue sauce can add a lot of sodium to your meals.

3. Baker's Items

Bread and rolls: Some commercial bread products are heavy in sodium, which adds to daily intake.

Pastries and baked goods frequently incorporate additional salt for flavor.

4. Cheese, Dairy Products

Processed Cheese: Cheese spreads and processed cheese slices contain more salt.

Cottage cheese is a healthful dairy alternative; however certain versions may have additional salt.

5. Meat & Deli Products

Processed Meats: Bacon, sausages, and deli meats are known for high salt levels.

Cured and smoked meats are frequently preserved using salt-based methods.

6. Snack foods

Salted Nuts and Seeds: Although nuts and seeds are healthful, salted variations increase sodium intake.

Potato chips and pretzels: Popular snack foods are frequently heavy in sodium for flavor.

7. Fast foods and restaurant dishes

French fries: Fast food items are notorious for their high salt content, with fries playing a big role.

Pizza, with its cheese, processed meats, and crust, can be a high-sodium option.

8. Instant and Packaged Foods

Instant noodles and pasta: Convenient alternatives frequently include high sodium spice packets.

Packaged Rice and Pasta Mixes: Pre-packaged convenience foods may include high salt content.

9. Pickled & Fermented Foods.

Pickles are high in sodium because of the pickling process.

Olives: Although healthful, olives can be heavy in sodium, especially when brined.

10. Certain beverages

Regular Soda: Regular sodas, which are often disregarded, can increase daily sodium intake.

Sports drinks: Although intended for hydration, they may contain additional sodium.

Strategies for Salt Reduction

Read Labels: Always check food labels for salt content. Select goods branded "low-sodium" or "sodium-free."

Choose Fresh, Whole Foods: Fresh fruits, vegetables, lean meats, and whole grains are inherently low in salt.

Cook at Home: Cooking meals at home gives you more control over the ingredients and sodium content.

Use Herbs and Spices: Instead of using salt, add flavor with herbs, spices, and other seasonings.

Limit Restaurant and Fast Food: When dining out, be aware of menu alternatives and request lower-sodium options or changes.

Gradual Reduction: Reduce the amount of salt in recipes gradually to allow the taste receptors to adjust to the decreased sodium levels.

Understanding the impact of high-sodium diets and making informed decisions is critical to overall health. Adopting a low-sodium diet can help prevent cardiovascular disease, kidney difficulties, and promote a healthy lifestyle.

Foods high in potassium and phosphorus

It is critical to balance potassium and phosphorus consumption, particularly for people who are managing kidney-related diseases such as Chronic Kidney Disease (CKD). Potassium is an essential mineral that regulates a variety of body functions, including muscle contractions and fluid equilibrium. Excess potassium intake, on the other hand, can be harmful to persons with impaired kidney function. Phosphorus, on the other hand, is essential for bone health, but high levels might be problematic for people who have kidney problems. Here's a complete review of foods rich in potassium and phosphorus.

Foods High in Potassium

1) Fruits

Bananas: Rich in potassium, bananas are a practical and portable supply of this crucial mineral.

Oranges: Citrus fruits, especially oranges, are high in potassium and have numerous health advantages.

2) Vegetables

Leafy Greens: Spinach, kale, and Swiss chard are high-potassium options.

Potatoes: Baked potatoes with skin are high in potassium.

3. Dairy and dairy alternatives.

Plain, low-fat, or Greek yogurt is a potassium-rich dairy product.

Milk contains potassium, as do fortified plant-based substitutes.

4. Legumes

Kidney Beans: Beans, especially kidney beans, are high in potassium.

Lentils include potassium, protein, and fiber.

5. Fish

Salmon: Fatty fish, such as salmon, are high in potassium and contain omega-3 fatty acids.

6. Nuts and seeds.

Pistachios: Nuts like pistachios are high in potassium and include healthful fats.

Sunflower seeds are a potassium-rich snack.

7. Meat

Lean meats such as chicken and turkey have moderate amounts of potassium.

Pork loin and tenderloin are potassium-rich alternatives.

8. Sweet potatoes

Sweet potatoes are nutrient-packed, providing potassium as well as other vitamins and fiber.

9. Avocado

Avocado is a creamy, potassium-rich fruit that also contains beneficial monounsaturated fats.

Foods Rich in Phosphorus

1. Dairy and dairy alternatives.

Dairy and fortified plant-based milk replacements are good sources of phosphorus.

Cheese: Hard and processed cheeses have greater phosphorus levels.

2. Meat and poultry.

Beef and pork: Red meats might increase phosphorus consumption.

Organ Meats: Liver and other organ meats are particularly phosphorus-rich.

3. Fish

Salmon is a good source of omega-3s, but it also includes phosphorus.

Sardines: Canned sardines are high in phosphorus and calcium.

4. Poultry

Chicken and turkey: Phosphorus is found in poultry, particularly dark meat.

5. Legumes

Lentils and beans are high in protein and fiber but also contain phosphorus.

Phosphorus can be found in soybean products such as tempeh and tofu.

6. Nuts and seeds.

Pumpkin Seeds: Seeds, including pumpkin seeds, might increase phosphorus intake.

Almonds: Nuts, including almonds, contain phosphorus.

7. Whole Grains

Whole wheat, like other whole grains, contributes to phosphorus intake.

Quinoa: While quinoa is a nutritious grain, it includes phosphorus.

8. Processed foods.

Processed foods like bacon, sausages, and deli meats may contain additional phosphorus.

Convenience Foods: Instant noodles and certain packaged foods may be rich in phosphorus.

Considerations for a Balanced Diet:

Portion Control.

Portion control helps to manage overall nutritional consumption, including potassium and phosphorus.

Balance and moderation

A kidney-friendly diet requires a mix of high-potassium and high-phosphorus foods.

Consult with healthcare professionals.

Individuals with kidney-related disorders should consult with healthcare specialists, particularly dietitians, for specialized dietary advice.

Individualized Approaches.

Dietary demands vary, and it is critical to customize dietary choices based on individual health, stage of kidney disease, and other considerations.

Regular Monitoring

Regular monitoring of blood levels and kidney function aids in determining the effect of dietary choices on potassium and phosphorus levels.

Understanding and regulating potassium and phosphorus consumption is critical for those with kidney problems. A balanced approach to nutrition, which includes a variety of foods and takes into account individual health needs, promotes general well-being while meeting specific dietary demands.

Processed and packaged foods

Processed and packaged foods are common in modern diets, providing convenience and shelf stability. However, the widespread consumption of these foods has generated concerns about their excessive levels of added sugars, harmful fats, sodium, and artificial ingredients. Understanding the effects of processed and packaged foods on health is critical for making sound dietary decisions. Here's a thorough examination of processed and packaged foods.

Features of Processed and Packaged Foods:

1. Additives and preservatives

Many processed foods contain artificial additives and preservatives that improve flavor, texture, and shelf life.

2. Refined ingredients.

Processed foods frequently employ refined components such as white flour and sugar, which deplete nutrients found in natural meals.

3. Unhealthy fats

Processed meals often include trans fats and high levels of saturated fat, which contribute to cardiovascular problems.

4. High sugar content.

Packaged goods, particularly candies, cereals, and beverages, sometimes include high levels of added sugars, which have an impact on metabolic health.

5. Sodium Concerns

Processed foods, such as snacks, canned soups, and ready meals, are rich in sodium, which can lead to hypertension and other health issues.

6. Reduced nutrient density.

Food nutrient density is often reduced during processing, resulting in a loss of vital vitamins, minerals, and fiber.

7. Convenience & Accessibility

Processed and packaged foods are appealing to people who lead busy lives because they are convenient and easy to get.

Examples of processed and packaged foods:

1. Snack food.

Chips: Potato chips, corn chips, and other snacks are frequently heavy in harmful fats and salt.

Sweets and candies are often loaded with extra sugars and artificial flavors.

2. Breakfast cereals

Many commercial cereals include a lot of sugar and may lack the critical elements present in whole grains.

3. Frozen meals.

Frozen dinners and entrees are generally rich in sodium and may lack the nutritional balance of home-cooked meals.

4. Canned soups

Canned soups are convenient, but they are typically rich in sodium, increasing overall salt intake.

5. Instant noodles and pasta.

These goods are convenient for quick meals, but they can be high in sodium and low in nutritional content.

6. Processed meats.

Hot dogs and sausages: Processed meats are notorious for their high salt and harmful fat levels.

Bacon is a processed meat that should be consumed in moderation due to its high saturated fat and salt content.

7. Sugary beverages.

Sodas: Carbonated beverages are known for their high sugar content.

Fruit juices and flavored drinks may have additional sugar.

8. Baker's Items

Many baked foods, including cookies, cakes, and pastries, contain high levels of refined sugars and harmful fats.

Health implications

1. Weight Gain and Obesity.

Many manufactured foods have high energy density, which can lead to overeating and weight gain.

2. Cardiovascular Issues.

Processed foods high in harmful fats and sodium can raise the risk of heart disease and hypertension.

3. Metabolic health.

Excessive consumption of added sugars in processed foods can lead to insulin resistance and metabolic problems.

4. Nutritional Deficiency

Relying on processed foods may lead to nutrient deficiencies, as they frequently lack vital vitamins, minerals, and fiber.

5. Digestive Health.

Low-fiber processed foods can cause digestive problems, including constipation.

Tips for Healthy Eating:

1. Read labels.

Check the ingredient list and nutrition label for added sugars, bad fats, and sodium levels.

2. Cook at home.

Preparing meals at home gives you more control over the materials and reduces your dependency on manufactured foods.

3. Choose whole foods.

Prioritize whole, minimally processed foods such as fruits and vegetables, lean meats, and whole grains.

4. Limit sugary drinks.

Choose water, herbal teas, or unsweetened beverages instead of sugary sodas and energy drinks.

5. Snack mindfully.

Choose whole food snacks such as fruits, nuts, and vegetables over processed snacks.

6. Moderation.

While the occasional use of processed foods is permissible, moderation is essential for a balanced and healthy diet.

Understanding the effects of processed and packaged foods on health is critical for making sound dietary decisions. While convenience is an obvious advantage, choosing whole, nutrient-dense foods is critical for long-term well-being and preventing the different health problems connected with processed food overconsumption.

Portion Control and Meal Planning

Navigating a healthy lifestyle entails not just selecting nutritious foods, but also practicing conscious portion control and intelligent meal planning. These habits have a significant impact on weight management, dietary balance, and general health. Portion control emphasizes the significance of limiting food consumption to avoid overeating, which aids in weight control and digestion. These practices, when combined with meal planning, which includes careful meal preparation and organization, promote healthy eating patterns. Meal planning not only assures a well-balanced diet, but it also helps you avoid making impulsive, less nutritious choices. This section sets the foundation for a full discussion of the advantages and practical tactics connected with portion control and meal planning, empowering individuals to make informed decisions for continued health and vitality.

Portion control is essential for keeping a healthy and balanced lifestyle. Portion management is an essential component of mindful eating, which is controlling the amount of food ingested during meals and snacks. Here's a thorough examination of the importance of portion control:

1. Weight Management.

Weight management relies heavily on portion control. Individuals can better regulate their calorie intake by adjusting their portion sizes, which can help with weight loss or maintenance.

2. Caloric Awareness

Controlling portion sizes increases awareness of caloric intake. Understanding the energy level of meals allows people to make more informed nutritional choices.

3. Blood Sugar Regulation

Balanced serving sizes help keep blood sugar levels constant. Consistent and moderate food intake helps reduce blood glucose spikes and crashes, which is especially important for diabetics.

4. Digestive Health.

Overeating can strain the digestive system, causing discomfort and problems such as indigestion. Portion control promotes efficient digestion and nutrition absorption.

5. Nutrient Distribution.

Smaller, more balanced portions provide for a more even distribution of key nutrients throughout the day, ensuring that the body receives an adequate supply of vitamins, minerals, and other vital components.

6. Prevents Overconsumption

Larger portions frequently result in overconsumption of calories, which contributes to weight gain and other health problems. Portion control can help you avoid consuming too many calories.

7. Cognitive Awareness.

Practicing portion control encourages mindfulness during meals. Being present and focused on the act of eating promotes a healthier connection with food.

8. Supports Metabolism

Eating smaller, more balanced meals can help maintain a constant metabolism. Regular and modest meals allow the body to efficiently use and burn calories.

9. Adaptable to dietary goals.

Portion control is adaptive to a variety of dietary goals, including weight loss, muscle building, and specific nutritional requirements. It offers a flexible approach to achieving individual health goals.

10. Teach Sustainable Habits

Developing portion management practices teaches long-term abilities for eating healthfully. It is a realistic and long-lasting approach to nutrition.

11. Prevents food waste.

Portion management lowers the possibility of making or ordering excess food, reducing food waste and increasing sustainability.

12. Enhances satisfaction.

Consuming suitable portions ensures that meals are satisfying but not unduly restricted. Feeling satiated after a meal promotes general well-being and adherence to a balanced eating routine.

Strategies for Effective Portion Control.

Use Smaller Plates: Choose smaller plates to give a fuller appearance with lesser amounts.

Practice Mindful Eating: Pay attention to hunger and fullness signs while eating deliberately and appreciating each bite.

Measure and Weigh Foods: Use measuring instruments to correctly determine portion proportions, especially when cooking at home.

Divide Restaurant Portions: When dining out, consider sharing plates or immediately portioning half for takeout.

Be Aware of Snacking: Pre-portion snacks into small containers to prevent thoughtless munching.

Include a Variety of Foods: A diversified diet with adequate quantities of different food categories promotes complete nutritional intake.

Stay Hydrated: Drinking water before meals will help you control your appetite and avoid overeating.

Plan Ahead: Use meal planning to prepare properly portioned meals and snacks in advance.

Portion control is an essential component of a healthy lifestyle, affecting weight management, nutritional balance, and general well-being. Individuals can create a long-term and healthy relationship with food by practicing mindful eating habits and knowing the value of portion sizes.

Tips for effective meal planning

Effective meal planning can help you maintain a balanced diet, save time, and improve your overall health. It requires careful planning, organization, and consideration of nutritional requirements. Here's a thorough examination of strategies for good meal planning:

1. Set clear objectives.

Define your goals, whether they are weight loss, improved nutrition, or time savings. Clear goals influence your food planning decisions.

2. Create a weekly schedule.

Plan your meals for the coming week, taking into account your daily activities, work schedules, and social responsibilities. A weekly routine simplifies grocery shopping and meal preparation.

3. Consider nutritional balance.

Each meal should have a healthy balance of macronutrients (carbohydrates, proteins, and fats) and micronutrients (vitamins and minerals). Include a range of dietary groups to ensure complete nourishment.

4. Choose whole, unprocessed foods:

Prioritize natural foods over processed ones. Fresh fruits and vegetables, lean proteins, and whole grains are rich in important nutrients and contain no preservatives or dangerous additives.

5. Prep Ingredients in Advance

Wash, cut, and portion the ingredients ahead of time. Having prepared foods on hand makes cooking faster and more convenient on hectic days.

6. Embrace batch cooking

Cook big quantities of staple foods such as cereals, meats, and sauces that may be used in several meals throughout the week. This saves time while ensuring consistent meal proportions.

7. Provide a variety of flavors and textures.

Make meals more pleasurable by combining different flavors and textures. To keep things interesting, try different herbs, spices, and cooking methods.

8. Plan for leftovers.

Cook additional amounts to have leftovers for lunch or dinner the following day. This reduces the requirement for ongoing meal preparation.

9. Be mindful of portion sizes.

Consider portion proportions to avoid overeating. Use measurement instruments or visual cues to estimate the proper portions for your nutritional goals.

10. Create Theme Nights.

Assign distinct themes to different days of the week (for example, Meatless Monday, Taco Tuesday) to add diversity and make meal planning easier.

11. Rotate staples.

Rotate staple foods such as grains, proteins, and vegetables to maintain a varied nutrient intake and avoid mealtime monotony.

12. Plan for flexibility.

Allow for flexibility and spontaneity. If your plans change or you want to try something new, be flexible with your meal planning method.

13. Utilize Leftover Ingredients

To reduce food waste and make the best use of your kitchen resources, plan the following meals around leftover items.

14. Take Advantage of Seasonal Produce

Include seasonal fruits and vegetables to increase freshness, flavor, and nutritional value. Seasonal vegetables are often less expensive and benefit local farmers.

15. Create a Shopping List

Prepare a detailed shopping list based on your food plan. Stick to the list to avoid impulse purchases and ensure you have all of the materials on hand.

16. Use technology.

Use meal planning applications or online tools to organize recipes, create grocery lists, and speed up the planning process.

17. Rotate Recipes

To avoid culinary boredom, keep a repertoire of favorite recipes while introducing new ones regularly.

18. Listen to Your Body

Pay attention to hunger and fullness signs. Adjust your meal plan to meet your body's demands and tastes.

19. Stay hydrated.

Remember to include hydration in your meal plan. Water, herbal teas, and other low-calorie liquids are all necessary components of a healthy diet.

20. Review and reflect

Regularly examine your meal planning strategy. Consider what worked well and what may be improved, and make any adjustments.

Successful meal planning is a dynamic and individualized process that promotes health, saves time, and makes meals more enjoyable. Individuals who incorporate these guidelines can create a durable and adaptable meal planning practice that is consistent with their lifestyle and nutritional goals.

Monitoring and Adjusting the Renal Diet

Monitoring and changing the renal diet is an important part of maintaining kidney function, especially for people with chronic kidney disease (CKD). This procedure entails closely monitoring food choices, hydration intake, and critical nutritional components to maintain optimal kidney function and general well-being. Here's a full look at monitoring and changing the renal diet:

1. Regular Dietary Assessments.

Regular dietary assessments assist individuals and healthcare providers in understanding how the renal diet affects kidney function. Monitoring entails assessing meal options, quantity quantities, and adherence to dietary rules.

2. Fluid Intake Monitoring

Tracking fluid consumption is critical, especially for people who have kidney difficulties. Maintaining an optimum fluid intake-to-output ratio helps to prevent fluid retention and electrolyte abnormalities.

3. Electrolyte levels

Regular blood tests measure electrolyte levels, such as potassium, phosphorus, and salt. Based on the test results, changes to the renal diet may be required to avoid imbalances that could strain the kidneys.

4. Protein Monitoring.

Protein consumption is an important concern in the renal diet. Regular monitoring ensures that those with kidney issues are getting enough high-quality protein without overburdening their kidneys.

5. Blood Pressure Management.

Monitoring blood pressure is crucial for kidney health. To help maintain blood pressure levels, the renal diet may be modified, for as by limiting sodium intake.

6. Urine Tests

Periodic urine testing can provide information on kidney function. Monitoring parameters such as proteinuria and urine concentration can assist in determining the success of the renal diet in maintaining kidney health.

7. Adjusting Sodium Intake

Sodium levels affect blood pressure and fluid balance. Individuals may need to change their salt intake based on their blood pressure and overall health.

8. Individualized Dietary Plans

Renal diets should be tailored to the stage of renal disease, underlying health problems, and individual dietary preferences. Regular assessments enable changes to meet changing needs.

9. Monitoring Medication Interactions.

Some drugs may interact with specific foods or nutrients. Regular monitoring ensures that the renal diet is compatible with prescription drugs, allowing adjustments to be made as needed.

10. Educating and Empowering Individuals

Educating people about the need for self-monitoring allows them to take an active role in their kidney health. This includes comprehending nutritional labels, controlling portion sizes, and making informed food choices.

11. Collaborating with Healthcare Professionals

Regular communication with healthcare specialists, such as nutritionists and nephrologists, is vital. Collaborative efforts enable continuous monitoring, adjustment, and optimization of the renal diet.

12. Adapting to Changing Conditions

Kidney function might change over time. The renal diet should be adaptive to changing health situations, meeting nutritional needs while reducing stress on the kidneys.

13. Maintaining a Food Diary

Keeping a food diary makes it easier to track and detect dietary patterns. Individuals can monitor their dietary and fluid intake, making it easier to discover areas for improvement.

14. Assessing Nutritional Deficiencies

Regular assessments help to identify any nutritional inadequacies. Adjustments to the renal diet can then be made to meet specific nutrient requirements, such as supplementation or diet adjustments.

15. Behavioral and lifestyle considerations

Monitoring goes beyond food choices and includes behavioral and lifestyle aspects. Stress, physical exercise, and sleep patterns are all factors to consider when approaching kidney health holistically.

16. Promoting Long-Term Adherence.

Regular monitoring and changes are intended to promote long-term adherence to the renal diet. Sustainability is critical to providing continued support for renal health.

17. Involving Support Systems

Involving family members and support networks in the monitoring process promotes a cooperative approach.

Individuals who must adhere to renal dietary limitations require a supportive atmosphere.

18. Celebrating Progress.

Recognizing and applauding beneficial dietary changes and adhering to the renal diet helps people stay motivated and devoted to their kidney health.

19. Staying Informed

Keeping up with the latest research and discoveries in renal nutrition enables ongoing improvement in dietary plans. Education enables people to make educated judgments.

20. Seeking professional advice

Individuals should seek professional advice if they have any problems or questions about their renal diet. Dietitians and healthcare professionals can provide individualized advice and make necessary changes.

Monitoring and changing the renal diet are continual activities that necessitate collaboration among patients, healthcare providers, and support systems. Regular examinations, adaptability to changing situations, and a proactive attitude to kidney health all help to increase the renal diet's effectiveness in supporting overall well-being.

Regular check-ups with healthcare professionals are an essential component of preventive healthcare, giving a proactive approach to maintaining overall health and addressing specific health concerns. These routine appointments include exams, screenings, and discussions with healthcare experts to evaluate health status, identify potential problems early on, and personalize interventions to individual requirements. Here's a thorough examination of the significance and elements of frequent check-ups:

1. Establishing a baseline.

Regular checkups serve to set a baseline for an individual's health. Vital signs, blood pressure, cholesterol levels, and other important health markers are all part of the baseline data.

2. Early Detection of Health Issues

Routine screenings and testing performed at check-ups aid in the early diagnosis of health problems. Identifying problems early on enables more effective and less invasive therapies.

3. Monitoring chronic conditions.

Individuals with chronic diseases such as diabetes, hypertension, or kidney disease require regular check-ups. Healthcare professionals can monitor illness development, change medications, and offer continuing support.

4. Immunization and Preventive Measures

Check-ups are used by healthcare providers to confirm that individuals have received all necessary vaccines and preventive measures. This is especially important for preventing infectious diseases and improving public health.

5. Medication Management.

Check-ups enable healthcare experts to assess and adjust drugs based on changes in health, adverse effects, or the need for further prescriptions.

6. Lifestyle and Behavioral Discussions

Healthcare providers do regular check-ups to examine lifestyle issues such as nutrition, physical exercise, and sleep patterns. These discussions assist individuals in making educated health-related decisions.

7. Mental Health Assessment.

Mental health is an important aspect of overall well-being. Regular check-ups allow for discussions about mental health concerns, stressors, and coping techniques, which can lead to appropriate interventions.

8. Comprehensive physical examinations.

Physical examinations during check-ups enable healthcare providers to evaluate a variety of body systems, including the cardiovascular, respiratory, and musculoskeletal.

9. Dental and Vision Check-ups

Regular dental and vision check-ups, while not typically included in general health screenings, are critical for preserving oral and optical health.

10. Blood Tests and Laboratory Screenings

Blood testing and laboratory screens are frequent parts of routine checkups. These tests can reveal important information regarding cholesterol levels, blood sugar, kidney function, and other vital indicators.

11. Health Risk Assessment.

Healthcare providers do health risk assessments to analyze lifestyle habits, family medical history, and other factors that may influence an individual's overall health risk.

12. Health Education and Promotion

Check-ups serve as opportunities for health education and promotion. Healthcare practitioners can advise on preventive measures, healthy practices, and resources for additional education.

13. Establishing Trust and Communication

Regular check-ups help to create trust between patients and their healthcare professionals. Open communication increases the efficacy of healthcare interventions.

14. Age and gender-specific screenings

During frequent check-ups, individuals may receive particular screenings and interventions based on their age and gender, such as mammograms, Pap smears, or prostate exams.

15. Managing Health Transitions.

Regular check-ups help manage health changes at all phases of life, from childhood and adolescence to adulthood and the elderly. Healthcare professionals can change care plans to meet changing needs.

16. Continuity of Care

Regular check-ups help to maintain continuity of care by allowing healthcare practitioners to track changes over time and verify that interventions are in line with long-term health goals.

17. Holistic Approach to Health

Check-ups support a holistic approach to health by considering physical, mental, and emotional well-being. This thorough approach promotes a more full picture of a person's health situation.

18. Identifying Health Disparities.

Regular healthcare visits help identify and resolve health inequities, ensuring that all people receive appropriate and equitable care.

19. Facilitating Timely Referrals

If particular health concerns are discovered during a check-up, healthcare providers can make prompt recommendations to experts for additional examination and treatment.

20. Empowering Individuals for Self-Care

Regular check-ups encourage people to take an active role in their health. Individuals may make informed decisions and practice good self-care habits with the help of education and assistance.

Regular check-ups with healthcare specialists are essential for preserving and enhancing health throughout one's lifetime. These consultations provide a complete approach to preventative care, early diagnosis of health issues, and continuous assistance for persons seeking to manage their entire well-being.

Making modifications based on individual health needs is an important part of customized healthcare, as it ensures that interventions, treatments, and lifestyle recommendations are matched to each person's specific needs. This approach acknowledges that people's health circumstances, genetic variables, lifestyle choices, and tastes vary greatly. Here's a thorough examination of the significance and components of making changes depending on individual health needs:

1. Personalized Treatment Plans

Individual health demands differ, and a personalized approach enables healthcare experts to create custom treatment regimens. This comprises drug regimes, therapies, and other interventions tailored to the individual health condition and its subtleties.

2. Genetic considerations

Genetic factors have a substantial impact on health. Genetic adjustments can help guide therapy decisions, pharmaceutical responses, and risk evaluations for specific illnesses.

3. Lifestyle and Behavioral Adjustments

Understanding your lifestyle choices and behavioral patterns is critical. Personalized adjustments may include suggestions for specific dietary changes, exercise regimens, stress management approaches, and sleep hygiene practices.

4. Chronic Disease Management

Chronic illnesses, such as diabetes, cardiovascular disease, and autoimmune disorders, may necessitate continuing management. Healthcare providers frequently analyze individual health needs and change treatment programs to improve management and quality of life.

5. Adapting to Changing Health Conditions

Health issues might change over time. Making adjustments based on changes in symptoms, illness progression, or therapy responses ensures that patients receive the most effective and up-to-date care.

6. Medication Tailoring

Medication regimens are modified based on individual responses, side effects, and changing health conditions. This ensures that medications are effective, well-tolerated, and in line with the patient's overall health objectives.

7. Customized Nutritional Guidance

Nutrition is extremely important in maintaining overall health. Personalized changes can include altering dietary advice to meet specific nutritional shortages, manage chronic disorders, or suit personal preferences and limits.

8. Mental Health Considerations

Mental health requirements are very individualized. Therapeutic techniques, counseling strategies, or drugs may be adjusted based on the specifics of an individual's mental health condition and response to interventions.

9. Support for Aging

As people age, their health needs alter. Adjustments may be required to address age-related problems, change treatment programs, and give appropriate assistance in maintaining health and independence.

10. Fertility and Reproductive Health

Personalized modifications are critical in the field of reproductive health, taking into account fertility concerns, family planning goals, and individual responses to hormone therapy.

11. Prevention and Wellness Strategies

Individual health needs must be considered when developing preventative measures and wellness plans. This includes risk factors, family history, and lifestyle choices. This method is proactive, addressing potential health risks before they worsen.

12. Cultural and Social Considerations

Adjustments based on cultural and socioeconomic aspects are critical for culturally competent care. This includes acknowledging and respecting various cultural traditions, beliefs, and socioeconomic determinants of health.

13. Patient Preferences and Values

Respecting patient choices and values is essential while making modifications. Understanding an individual's objectives and aspirations enables healthcare providers to match interventions with what is most important to the individual.

14. Allergies and sensitivities.

Changes must be made to accommodate allergies and sensitivities to drugs, foods, or environmental variables. This guarantees that interventions are safe and do not result in unwanted effects.

15. Accessibility and affordability.

Making changes also requires taking into account practical concerns such as the accessibility and price of healthcare interventions. This guarantees that patients can follow suggested therapies without incurring unnecessary financial stress.

16. Continuous Monitoring and Assessment

Regular monitoring and assessment of individual health requirements is required. This entails continual communication between healthcare practitioners and patients to track progress, address developing problems, and adjust care plans accordingly.

17. Patient Empowerment.

Empowering patients to actively participate in their care promotes a collaborative approach. Education, including people in decision-making, and appreciating their contributions all help to make more effective changes.

18. Timely Referrals and Consultations

When changes necessitate specific expertise, healthcare providers make prompt recommendations to specialists or consultants. This guarantees that people receive complete, competent treatment for their specific health needs.

19. Communication and Shared Decision-Making

Open communication and shared decision-making are critical in making changes. Informed interactions between healthcare practitioners and patients help them navigate treatment alternatives, potential hazards, and the reasoning behind changes.

20. Holistic and Integrative Approaches

Individuals' holistic needs are addressed by integrating physical, mental, and social elements of health. To attain holistic well-being, adjustments may include implementing collaborative care models, including complementary therapies, and addressing societal determinants.

Making modifications to meet individual health needs is a dynamic and ongoing process. It necessitates a personalized, patient-centered approach that respects each individual's individuality and seeks to improve health outcomes by personalizing interventions to their specific needs.

CHAPTER THREE

SMOOTHIE CLEANSER GUIDE

Navigating a renal diet with an emphasis on cleansing and nourishing, the Smoothie Cleanser Guide becomes an invaluable resource for people maintaining kidney health. This part, tailored to the specific nutritional needs of renal care, presents a step-by-step strategy for creating smoothies that not only entice the taste senses but also encourage kidney-friendly nutrition. It delves into the world of renal health-promoting foods, revealing a variety of flavors and nutrients that have been carefully selected to enhance kidney function. Whether you're on a renal diet or looking for a new approach to nourishing your kidneys, this section combines creativity and utility, making the path to renal fitness both entertaining and nutritious.

Introduction to Smoothie Cleansing

Exploring creative approaches to nutrition is common when embarking on a quest to improve overall well-being, and

Smoothie Cleansing is one such route that is becoming increasingly popular. This holistic and refreshing approach goes beyond standard diets, delivering a nutritional blend of whole-food ingredients in a simple, sippable format. Smoothie cleaning combines the benefits of nutrient-dense fruits, vegetables, and other healthy ingredients to detoxify the body, increase energy, and enhance overall health.

Key Ingredients of Smoothie Cleansing

1. Nutrient-Rich Ingredients

Smoothie cleaning depends on the nutritional value of fresh fruits, leafy greens, super foods, and plant-based proteins. These substances contain critical vitamins, minerals, and antioxidants that are necessary for overall health.

2. Hydration and detoxification.

Smoothies' high water content promotes hydration, while natural detoxifying chemicals help the body's cleansing processes. This dual action helps to eliminate pollutants while also promoting a healthy interior environment.

3. Digestive Support.

Smoothies frequently contain fiber-rich components, which improve digestive health and promote a sense of fullness. This promotes weight management and nutrient absorption.

4. Convenient and customizable.

Smoothie cleansing provides a practical and personalized approach to nutrition. Individuals can customize their smoothies to fulfill specific dietary requirements, making them accessible to a variety of lifestyles and interests.

5. Sustainable Lifestyle Integration

Unlike fad diets, smoothie cleansing emphasizes long-term lifestyle changes. It promotes a healthy relationship with food by promoting the use of nutrient-dense ingredients in daily routines.

6. Flavorful and enjoyable

Smoothie cleaning is about more than just nourishing the body; it's also about pleasing the palate. The variety of flavors and textures make this method appealing, transforming nourishment into a delightful experience.

7. Balanced Nutritional Intake

Smoothie cleansing promotes balanced nutritional intake by offering a variety of key nutrients. This helps to treat any shortages while also promoting overall well-being.

How to Start Smoothie Cleansing

1. Ingredients Selection

Depending on your dietary preferences and health goals, select a selection of fresh fruits, leafy greens, vegetables, and other ingredients such as nuts, seeds, or dairy alternatives.

2. Blender Mastery

Invest in a high-quality blender to achieve a smooth and consistent texture. This equipment is essential for breaking down fibrous components and maximizing nutritional benefits.

3. Recipe Exploration

Explore different smoothie recipes to find combinations that fit your tastes. Incorporate health-promoting components, such as berries for antioxidants and spinach for iron.

4. Meal replacement or supplement.

Smoothie cleansing can be used as a meal replacement or as an addition to current meals, giving you more flexibility in incorporating it into your routine.

5. Hydration Emphasis

Include liquid bases such as water, coconut water, or herbal teas in your smoothies to increase hydration. Hydrating elements aid in the cleansing and rejuvenation process.

6. Gradual integration.

Start by gradually incorporating smoothie cleanses into your daily regimen. This allows the body to adjust and provides an opportunity to evaluate how it improves energy levels and overall well-being.

Smoothie cleansing, as an accessible and fun approach to eating, combines health and enjoyment. With an emphasis on nutrient-dense ingredients and tailored flexibility, this practice allows people to embark on a journey of nourishment, vigor, and the joy of savoring each drink on the path to a healthy existence.

Benefits of incorporating smoothies into the diet

Blending smoothies into your diet is a delicious and nutritious method to improve overall health. Smoothies provide numerous benefits, ranging from increased food consumption to greater hydration and convenience. Here's a complete look at the benefits of making smoothies a regular part of your diet:

1. Nutrient Density

Smoothies provide a concentrated dose of nutrients by blending fruits, vegetables, and other healthy components in one delightful drink. This encourages appropriate nutrient intake, which is necessary for general health.

2. Increased fruit and vegetable consumption.

Smoothies are a practical and enjoyable option for people who struggle to eat enough fruits and vegetables. Blending allows you to combine many servings into a single, easy-to-drink serving.

3. Hydration Support.

Many smoothie recipes include hydrating ingredients like water-rich fruits and vegetables, which add to overall hydration. This is especially helpful for people who struggle to satisfy their daily hydration needs.

4. Digestive Health & Fiber Intake

Smoothies' fiber content, which comes from fruits, vegetables, and other plant-based ingredients, promotes digestive health. Adequate fiber intake supports regular bowel movements and healthy gut microbiota.

5. Quick and convenient.

Smoothies are a time-saving and convenient choice for busy people. They can be prepared in minutes and are an excellent choice for a nutritious breakfast, snack, or on-the-go meal replacement.

6. Versatility in Ingredients

Smoothies' adaptability allows for more creative component combinations. From leafy greens and almonds to yogurt and seeds, the options are limitless. This versatility guarantees that smoothies can be tailored to individual taste preferences and dietary requirements.

7. Weight Management

Including smoothies in a balanced diet can support weight management. The fiber and water content adds to a sense of fullness, which may reduce overall calorie consumption and aid in weight management.

8. Improved nutrient absorption.

Blending ingredients in a smoothie breaks down cell membranes, making nutrients more readily available for absorption. This increases vitamin and mineral bioavailability, allowing the body to use them more efficiently.

9. Energy Boost.

Natural sugars found in fruits provide an immediate source of energy. Smoothies can be a nutritious and invigorating pick-me-up, making them a perfect pre-or post-workout snack.

10. Customizable to Dietary Preferences

Smoothies are highly customisable to meet specific dietary needs and constraints. Whether you practice a vegetarian, vegan, or gluten-free diet, there are numerous options to suit your preferences.

11. Supports Skin Health

Nutrient-dense smoothie ingredients, such as antioxidants from berries and vitamins from fruits, help to maintain skin health. These elements help to prevent oxidative stress and support a healthy complexion.

12. Blood Sugar Control

Smoothies with protein, healthy fats, and fiber help to balance blood sugar levels. This might be especially advantageous for people with diabetes or who want to maintain their energy levels throughout the day.

13. Encourages Healthy Eating Habits

Smoothies promote a favorable attitude toward healthy eating. It's an exciting way to incorporate new fruits, veggies, and superfoods into your everyday diet.

14. Aids in Detoxification

Certain smoothie ingredients, such as leafy greens and citrus fruits, have purifying effects. They can help the body's natural detoxification processes and maintain a healthy interior environment.

15. Enhances Immune Function

Smoothies' high vitamin and antioxidant content might help build a strong immune system. Regular ingestion may help prevent infections and improve overall immune function.

16. Promotes Heart Health Many smoothies contain heart-healthy ingredients such as berries, oats, and almonds. These components may help decrease cholesterol and promote cardiovascular health.

17. Facilitates Nutritional Recovery

Smoothies can be a pleasant and healthy alternative for people who are recovering from illness or going through medical procedures. They give critical nutrients without causing undue stress on the digestive system.

Smoothies are an enticing technique to boost hydration in youngsters who may resist drinking plain water. Blending fruits and water produces a pleasant and hydrating beverage.

19. Eases Swallowing Difficulty

Smoothies are a more appealing and easy-to-consume option for people who have difficulties swallowing solid foods. This can be especially useful for the elderly or people with certain medical conditions.

20. Sustainable and environmentally friendly

Smoothies, particularly those made with local and seasonal ingredients, can help you make more sustainable and environmentally responsible eating choices. This is consistent with eco-conscious dietary practices.

The benefits of incorporating smoothies into your diet go beyond just delight. They are a versatile and pleasurable complement to a well-balanced diet, providing a variety of health advantages that contribute to general well-being.

Smoothies, which are vivid combinations of fruits, vegetables, and liquid delight, can help keep your kidneys healthy. Individuals with kidney issues can enjoy a pleasant and nutritious meal by tailoring smoothies to meet renal dietary recommendations. Here's an in-depth look at how smoothies might be useful allies in promoting kidney health:

1. Hydration reinforcement

Renal health depends on adequate hydration. Smoothies, which frequently contain water-rich fruits and vegetables, contribute to overall fluid intake. Adequate hydration promotes kidney function, aiding in the clearance of waste.

2. Kidney-Friendly Ingredients

Making smoothies with kidney-friendly components is essential. Selecting low-potassium fruits such as berries, apples, and pears, as well as including renal-friendly greens like as kale and spinach, offers a nutrient-dense blend without an overdose of potassium.

3. Controlled Phosphorus Intake

Phosphorus intake is frequently monitored in renal diets. Smoothies can be adjusted to contain ingredients with lower phosphorus concentrations, allowing people to enjoy a tasty beverage without jeopardizing their renal health.

4. Moderate Protein Inclusion.

Protein moderation is essential for renal health. Smoothies allow you to include controlled amounts of plant-based proteins such as tofu, chia seeds, or hemp seeds, which promote balanced protein consumption.

5. Antioxidant-Rich Choices

Antioxidants serve an important role in lowering oxidative stress, which can impair kidney function. Smoothies made with antioxidant-rich foods like blueberries, cranberries, and red bell peppers help to maintain a renal-friendly nutritional profile.

6. Dietary Fiber for Digestive Harmony

Renal-friendly smoothies frequently include fiber from fruits and vegetables, which promotes digestive health without overloading the body with potassium or phosphorus. Adequate fiber promotes regular bowel motions.

7. Fluid-Based Hydration Emphasis

Emphasizing hydrating liquid bases such as water, coconut water, or herbal teas in smoothies increases fluid intake. This not only promotes hydration but also helps to cleanse and revitalize the kidneys.

8. Balancing Electrolytes

Smoothies can help balance electrolytes. Ingredients with moderate potassium content, such as bananas, can be deliberately used to ensure a harmonious electrolyte balance that supports kidney health.

9. Emphasis on Low Sodium Choices

Renal diets frequently entail lowering salt intake. Smoothies enable people to avoid high-sodium ingredients, promoting a kidney-friendly approach that is consistent with the goal of salt reduction.

10. Promotion of Alkaline Balance

Some typical smoothie ingredients, such as leafy greens and some fruits, may help the body maintain an alkaline balance. This can be good for people who want to keep their surroundings more alkaline, which may help with kidney health.

11. Gentle on the Digestive System

Smoothies, being in liquid form, are naturally kinder on the digestive tract. For people with kidney problems, this can be beneficial because it provides a pleasant and easily digestible source of important nutrients.

12. Customizable to Dietary Restrictions

Renal-friendly smoothies are very customizable, allowing for adjustments to particular dietary limitations. This versatility guarantees that people with unique dietary demands can still enjoy a range of cuisines while adhering to their renal health requirements.

13. Encourage Healthy Snacking

Smoothies are a tasty and nutritious snack alternative. Incorporating kidney-friendly components makes smoothies a popular alternative for people trying to eat responsibly while addressing renal health.

14. Addressing Potential Micronutrient Deficiencies

Renal diets can sometimes lead to micronutrient deficits. Smoothies, with their broad component profiles, can help address these shortages by delivering a wide range of vital vitamins and minerals in an easily absorbable manner.

15. Enhanced Nutrient Absorption

Blending components in smoothies improves nutritional absorption by breaking down cell barriers. This can be especially advantageous for people with impaired kidney function, ensuring that they get the most nutritious value.

16. Supportive of Overall Well-Being

A well-balanced, renal-friendly smoothie can improve overall health. Smoothies become allies in the pursuit of holistic health by providing important nutrients to the body while also taking into account kidney health factors.

Crafting a Renal-Friendly Smoothie:

Creating a renal-friendly smoothie involves a thoughtful selection of ingredients. Consider using:

Low-potassium fruits include berries, apples, and pears.

Renal-friendly greens include kale and spinach.

Controlled phosphorus sources include almond milk and coconut water.

Tofu, chia seeds, and hemp seeds are moderate protein sources.

Antioxidant-rich options include blueberries, cranberries, and red bell peppers.

Hydrating bases include water, herbal teas, and coconut water.

Smoothies, when intelligently prepared, can become an essential component of a renal-friendly diet. By connecting components with renal health principles, people can enjoy these nutritious blends as part of their kidney health strategy. Consult a healthcare practitioner or a qualified dietitian for specialized dietary advice based on your specific health concerns.

Renal-Friendly Smoothie Recipes

Renal-friendly smoothie recipes are a tasty approach to improving kidney function. Incorporating nutrient-dense, low-potassium fruits such as berries and apples, as well as renal-friendly greens like kale, results in a tasty yet kidney-friendly blend. Choosing hydrated bases like water or herbal teas, as well as controlled protein sources like tofu or chia seeds, results in a refreshing cocktail suited for people watching their renal diet. These smoothies not only supply necessary nutrients, but they are also a delightful and hydrating choice for anyone looking to nourish their bodies while adhering to renal health guidelines.

Low-potassium and low-phosphorus ingredient options

Maintaining optimal kidney function frequently entails following a diet that limits potassium and phosphorus intake. For people with kidney problems, integrating low-potassium and low-phosphorus foods is essential. Let's take a comprehensive look at these dietary components:

Low-Potassium Ingredients:

1. Berries

Berries, such as strawberries, blueberries, and raspberries, are tasty low-potassium fruits high in antioxidants and fiber.

2. Apples.

Peeled apples make for a crisp, low-potassium snack. They are versatile and can be used in a variety of cuisines.

3. Cucumbers

Cucumbers are hydrating and low in potassium, making them an ideal complement to salads and smoothies.

4) Cabbage

Cabbage is a low-potassium cruciferous vegetable that can be used to stir-fries or served as coleslaw.

5) Cauliflower

Cauliflower is a flexible, low-potassium vegetable that may be substituted for rice or roasted to make a healthful side dish.

6. Rice

White rice is a low-potassium grain that may be used as a base for many meals while maintaining potassium levels.

7. Egg whites.

Egg whites are low in potassium and can be mixed into meals to provide a protein boost without the potassium found in the yolk.

8. Berries

Grapes, when in moderation, can be a low-potassium fruit alternative.

9. Cranberries

Cranberries, in their unsweetened form, can give a tart flavor to foods and beverages without containing too much potassium.

10. Choose strained fruit juices (e.g., apple or cranberry) instead of whole fruits for lower potassium intake.

Low-Phosphorus Ingredient Options

1. Rice Milk This dairy replacement is low in phosphorus, making it ideal for people watching their intake.

2. Olive Oil Olive oil is a low-phosphorus, heart-healthy fat that may be used for cooking and salads.

Egg whites are low in potassium and phosphorus, making them a great protein source.

4. Fresh herbs.

Fresh herbs such as parsley, cilantro, and basil contribute flavor to recipes without adding much phosphorus.

5. Cornstarch.

Cornstarch, employed as a thickening agent, is a low-phosphorus substitute for flour in cooking and baking.

6. Unsalted Popcorn Air-popped, unsalted popcorn is a low-phosphorus food that can fulfill crunch needs.

7. Rice & Rice Products

White rice and rice-based products are low in phosphorus and can serve as a staple in a kidney-friendly diet.

8. Cabbage

Cabbage is not only low in potassium but also low in phosphorus, making it suited for a variety of culinary applications.

9. Berries are an antioxidant-rich and low-phosphorus fruit, making them an excellent choice.

10. Nondairy Creamers

Some non-dairy creamer substitutes contain less phosphorus than traditional dairy, making them suitable for persons with dietary requirements.

Considerations for Renal-Friendly Eating

Portion Control: Even low-potassium and low-phosphorus foods should be consumed in moderation to provide a healthy diet.

Individual nutritional needs differ, thus consultation with healthcare specialists or a licensed dietitian is essential for tailored assistance.

Reading food labels: Paying attention to food labels might help you detect hidden potassium and phosphorus sources in packaged goods.

Diversifying the Diet: Including a variety of low-potassium and low-phosphorus meals promotes a balanced and enjoyable eating experience while also promoting renal health.

Navigating a renal-friendly diet necessitates mindfulness and dedication to choosing products that comply with potassium and phosphorus limits. Individuals with kidney issues can enjoy a rich and satisfying culinary adventure while improving overall renal health by adding these low-potassium and low-phosphorus options.

Making nutrient-dense smoothies for renal health necessitates careful ingredient selection that strikes a balance between flavor and kidney-friendliness. Individuals can enjoy delectable smoothies that promote renal function by adding low potassium and low phosphorus alternatives while focusing on critical nutrients. Let's take a complete look at nutrient-dense smoothie mixes intended exclusively for renal well-being:

1. Berrylicious Kidney Boost

Ingredients include blueberries, cranberries, red grapes, cucumber, spinach, and water.

Renal Considerations: Low in potassium and phosphorus but high in antioxidants, vitamins, and hydration support.

2. Peachy Green Renewal Ingredients

Peaches, Pineapple, Spinach, Coconut Water, Chia Seeds.

Renal considerations: Low in potassium and phosphorus; high in vitamins, fiber, and omega-3 fatty acids.

3. Cucumber Mint Refresher Ingredients: Cucumber, Mint Leaves, Lemon Juice, Berries, Almond Milk.

Renal Considerations: Low in potassium and phosphorus, but hydrated with a rush of pleasant flavors.

4. Watermelon Basil Splash Ingredients

Watermelon, Basil Leaves, Strawberries, Greek Yogurt, Water.

Renal Considerations: Low in potassium and phosphorus; provides hydration, vitamins, and a hint of cream.

5. Carrot Ginger Citrus Soother

Ingredients include carrot, orange, ginger, turmeric, and coconut water.

Renal Considerations: Low potassium and phosphorus content; anti-inflammatory effects, vitamins, and hydration.

6. Apple Cinnamon Delight Ingredients

Peeled apples, cinnamon, almond butter, flaxseeds, and rice milk.

Renal Considerations: Low in potassium and phosphorus; high in fiber, healthy fats, and a touch of warmth.

7. Melon Mint Cooler

Ingredients: Cantaloupe, Honeydew, Mint Leaves, Lime Juice, and Coconut Water.

Renal Considerations: Low in potassium and phosphorus; refreshing and high in vitamins.

8. Avocado Berry Fusion Ingredients include avocado, mixed berries, chia seeds, and almond milk.

Renal Considerations

Moderate potassium, low phosphorus; contains healthful fats, fiber, and antioxidants.

9. Vanilla Almond Cream Dream Ingredients

Almond Milk, Vanilla Extract, Banana, Cauliflower (frozen), Oats.

Renal Considerations: Low in potassium and phosphorus, but a creamy, healthy alternative.

10. Mango Turmeric Elixir Ingredients

Mango, Turmeric, Coconut Milk, Spinach, Hemp Seeds.

Renal Concerns: Low potassium and phosphorus content; anti-inflammatory, vitamin, and plant-based protein.** Tips for Renal Nutrient-Dense Smoothies:

Portion Control: Even with kidney-friendly substances, moderation is essential to avoid excessive nutrient consumption.

To maintain fluid balance, use hydrating bases such as water, coconut water, or herbal teas.

Balanced Nutrient Profile: To make a well-rounded smoothie, include carbohydrates, proteins, and healthy fats.

Adapt to nutritional Restrictions: Customize recipes to meet individual nutritional needs, and seek specialized advice from healthcare professionals.

Investigate Low-Potassium Options: Include fruits and vegetables with lower potassium levels to ensure renal health compatibility.

Limit your high-phosphorus choices: Be aware of phosphorus levels and choose ingredients that comply with phosphorus limitations.

Making nutrient-dense smoothies for renal health is a creative endeavor that entails balancing flavors, textures, and kidney-friendly factors. By combining the correct ingredients, people can enjoy tasty and nourishing smoothies that not only satisfy their taste buds but also help to support and maintain kidney health.

Maintaining a renal-friendly diet does not require compromising flavor. It is easy to add depth and interest to meals without jeopardizing kidney health by using herbs, spices, and low-potassium items carefully and creatively. Let's look at complete recommendations for introducing delicious flavors into a renal diet.

1. Herb elevation

Fresh herbs: Fresh herbs such as basil, mint, cilantro, and parsley can add a burst of flavor. They are low in potassium and can enhance the flavor of salads, sauces, and marinades.

Dry Herbs: Dried herbs like oregano, thyme, and rosemary can be sprinkled on foods for a concentrated flavor boost.

2. Citrus Zest Zing.

Use the zest of citrus fruits (lemon, lime, or orange) to enhance brightness without adding much potassium. Zest can be used in salad dressings, sauces, and desserts.

3. Vinegar Versatility.

To improve the flavors of salads and marinades, use various kinds of vinegar in moderation, such as balsamic or red wine. They offer taste without adding extra potassium.

4. Spice Spectrum.

Experiment with kidney-friendly spices like cumin, coriander, cinnamon, turmeric, and ginger to add warmth and richness to your foods. These spices are typically poor in potassium.

5. Onion and Garlic Magic.

Utilize the fragrant properties of onions and garlic. Use them as a basis in savory meals to provide depth without jeopardizing renal health.

6. Broths with low potassium

Use low-potassium broths or stocks to add savory tastes to soups, stews, and rice meals. Homemade broths offer greater control over the components.

7. Mustard Momentum.

To add a tangy kick to salads, marinades, or sauces, choose low-potassium mustard variants. Mustard is a tasty alternative to high-sodium condiments.

8. Berries add a sweet note.

Berries, like strawberries or blueberries, can offer a touch of sweetness to both savory and sweet recipes. They are lower in potassium than other fruits.

9. Pesto Prowess

Make pesto with kidney-friendly ingredients like basil, pine nuts, garlic, and Parmesan cheese (in moderation). Use it as a sauce or spread to flavor pasta, grilled meats, and veggies.

10. Tomato Transformation.

While fresh tomatoes may be limited due to their potassium concentration, consider low-potassium tomato alternatives such as sun-dried tomatoes or tomato paste for concentrated flavor.

11. Lemon and herb-infused oils

To make infused oils, combine low-potassium herbs with olive oil or other kidney-friendly oils. Drizzle over salads or use in a mild sauté.

12. Low-Potassium Salsas

Create salsas with kidney-friendly components such as onions, cilantro, and a limited amount of tomatoes. Use it as a protein topping or a vegetable dip.

13. Mushroom Marvel.

Use the umami-rich flavor of mushrooms to enhance savory recipes. Mushrooms are a great addition to soups and stir-fries and as a meat alternative.

14. Nuts and seeds

 To add texture and flavor to foods, sprinkle crushed, low-potassium nuts or seeds (such as almonds). Use them cautiously to limit phosphorus intake.

15. Coconut creations

 Incorporate coconut milk or shredded coconut in moderation for a tropical flair. Coconut can be used in both savory and sweet recipes.

16. Mindful Salt Usage

Use herbs and spices to lessen your need for salt. If necessary, choose herbs with low potassium, such as dill or chives, rather than high-sodium equivalents.

17. Homemade dressings

Make homemade dressings with kidney-friendly components such as olive oil, vinegar, mustard, and herbs. This gives you control over the sodium and potassium content.

18. Roasting Magic.

Roast veggies to bring forth their natural tastes. The caramelization process transforms ordinary veggies into delectable additions to your meals.

19. Dill Pickle Twist.

Add the tart, low-potassium flavor of dill pickles to recipes. For a distinct flavor, add them to salads or use them as a garnish.

20. Capitalize on Capers

Capers are low in potassium and provide a saline, sour flavor to foods. Add them to sauces, salads, or as a protein topper.

Considerations For Flavorful Renal Eating:

Individual Sensitivities: Pay attention to your specific tolerance and modify the components accordingly.

Consult with Healthcare Professionals: For personalized recommendations on renal-friendly flavor enhancement, speak with a healthcare expert or a qualified dietitian.

Experiment with Combinations: Be creative and try different flavor combinations to see what matches your tastes.

Control Portion Sizes: Even low-potassium and low-phosphorus items should be consumed in moderation to maintain a healthy renal diet.

Adding taste to a renal-friendly diet involves some experimentation and innovation. By implementing these suggestions, people can embark on a gastronomic journey that not only satisfies their taste senses but also promotes kidney health.

Sample smoothie recipes for renal health.

Creating a varied range of kidney-friendly smoothies requires careful ingredient selection to maintain flavor and nutritional balance. Here are 15 sample smoothie recipes that are not only delicious but also appropriate for renal health

1. Berry Blast Bonanza

Ingredients:

1/2 cup blueberries (fresh or frozen)

1/2 cup raspberries (fresh or frozen)

1/2 cup strawberries (fresh or frozen)

1/4 cup cranberries (unsweetened, frozen)

1 tablespoon chia seeds

1 cup water or coconut water

Instructions:

Blend all berries with chia seeds until smooth.

Adjust consistency with water or coconut water.

Pour into a glass and relish the antioxidant-rich goodness.

2. Pineapple Paradise Punch

Ingredients:

1 cup pineapple (fresh or frozen)

1/2 banana (fresh or frozen, peeled and sliced)

1/4 cup cucumber (peeled and sliced)

1 tablespoon flaxseeds

1 cup coconut water

Instructions:

Blend pineapple, banana, and cucumber until smooth.

Add flaxseeds and coconut water; blend again.

Pour into a glass and enjoy this tropical treat.

3. Mango Tango Infusion

Ingredients:

1 cup mango (fresh or frozen, peeled and diced)

1/2 cup strawberries (fresh or frozen)

1/4 cup avocado

1 tablespoon hemp seeds

1/4 teaspoon turmeric

1 cup almond milk

Instructions:

Blend mango, strawberries, and avocado until creamy.

Add hemp seeds, turmeric, and almond milk; blend again.

Pour into a glass and savor the tropical twist.

4. Citrus Sensation Symphony

Ingredients:

1/2 orange (peeled and segmented)

1/2 grapefruit (peeled and segmented)

1/2 cup cucumber (peeled and sliced)

1 tablespoon chia seeds

1/4 teaspoon ginger (freshly grated)

1 cup water or herbal tea

Instructions:

Blend orange, grapefruit, and cucumber until smooth.

Add chia seeds, ginger, and water or herbal tea; blend again.

Pour into a glass and relish the zesty and hydrating blend.

5. Green Goddess Revival

Ingredients:

1 cup spinach (fresh or frozen)

1/2 cup kale (fresh or frozen)

1/2 banana (fresh or frozen, peeled and sliced)

1 tablespoon chia seeds

1/4 cup Greek yogurt

1 cup water or coconut water

Instructions:

Blend spinach, kale, and banana until smooth.

Add chia seeds, Greek yogurt, and water or coconut water; blend again.

Pour into a glass and enjoy this green powerhouse.

6. Papaya Pleasure Fusion

Ingredients:

1 cup papaya (fresh or frozen, peeled and diced)

1/2 cup strawberries (fresh or frozen)

1/4 cup avocado

1 tablespoon flaxseeds

1 cup coconut water

Instructions:

Blend papaya, strawberries, and avocado until creamy.

Add flaxseeds and coconut water; blend again.

Pour into a glass and savor the tropical delight.

7. Kiwi Kaleidoscope Crush

Ingredients:

2 kiwis (peeled and sliced)

1 cup kale (fresh or frozen)

1/2 banana (fresh or frozen, peeled and sliced)

1 tablespoon chia seeds

1/4 cup almond butter

1 cup water or almond milk

Instructions:

Blend kiwis, kale, and banana until smooth.

Add chia seeds, almond butter, and water or almond milk; blend again.

Pour into a glass and relish this vibrant kiwi-kale fusion.

8. Blueberry Basil Bliss

Ingredients:

1/2 cup blueberries (fresh or frozen)

1/4 cup basil leaves

1/2 cup cucumber (peeled and sliced)

1 tablespoon chia seeds

1/4 cup Greek yogurt

1 cup water or coconut water

Instructions:

Blend blueberries, basil, and cucumber until smooth.

Add chia seeds, Greek yogurt, and water or coconut water; blend again.

Pour into a glass and enjoy the refreshing blueberry-basil infusion.

9. Strawberry Mint Marvel

Ingredients:

1 cup strawberries (fresh or frozen)

1/4 cup mint leaves

1/2 cucumber (peeled and sliced)

1 tablespoon chia seeds

1/4 teaspoon ginger (freshly grated)

1 cup water or herbal tea

Instructions:

Blend strawberries, mint, and cucumber until smooth.

Add chia seeds, ginger, and water or herbal tea; blend again.

Pour into a glass and relish the minty freshness.

10. Melon Medley Magic

Ingredients

1 cup cantaloupe (fresh or frozen, diced)

1/2 cup honeydew (fresh or frozen, diced)

1/2 cup watermelon (fresh or frozen, diced)

1 tablespoon flaxseeds

1/4 cup coconut milk

1 cup water

Instructions:

1. Blend cantaloupe, honeydew, and watermelon until smooth.

2. Add flaxseeds, coconut milk, and water; blend again.

3. Pour into a glass and savor the refreshing melon fusion.

11. Raspberry Rose Refresher

Ingredients:

half cup of raspberries, either fresh or frozen

1/4 cup rose water

1/2 cup cucumber (peeled and sliced)

1 tablespoon chia seeds

1/4 cup Greek yogurt

1 cup water or coconut water

Instructions:

1. Blend raspberries, rose water, and cucumber until smooth.

2. Add chia seeds, Greek yogurt, and water or coconut water; blend again.

3. Pour into a glass and enjoy the floral raspberry-rose infusion.

12. Cherry Almond Dream

Ingredients:

half cup cherries (fresh or frozen and pitted)

1/4 cup almonds (unsalted)

1/2 banana (fresh or frozen, peeled and sliced)

1 tablespoon flaxseeds

1/4 teaspoon cinnamon

1 cup almond milk

Instructions:

1. Blend cherries, almonds, and banana until creamy.

2. Add flaxseeds, cinnamon, and almond milk; blend again.

3. Pour into a glass and savor the cherry-almond goodness.

13. Apple Cinnamon Symphony

Ingredients:

1 cup apples (peeled, cored, and diced)

1/2 teaspoon cinnamon

1/4 cup oats (uncooked)

1/2 cup Greek yogurt

1 tablespoon chia seeds

1 cup water or almond milk

Instructions:

1. Blend apples and cinnamon until smooth.

2. Add oats, Greek yogurt, chia seeds, and water or almond milk; blend again.

3. Pour into a glass and enjoy the apple-cinnamon harmony.

14. Blackberry Basil Burst

Ingredients:

1/2 cup blackberries (fresh or frozen)

1/4 cup basil leaves

1/2 cup cucumber (peeled and sliced)

1 tablespoon chia seeds

1/4 cup coconut water

1/4 cup water

Instructions:

1. Blend blackberries, basil, and cucumber until smooth.

2. Add chia seeds, coconut water, and water; blend again.

3. Pour into a glass and relish the unique blackberry-basil fusion.

15. Carrot Cake Celebration

Ingredients:

1/2 cup carrots (peeled and sliced)

1/4 cup pineapple (fresh or frozen)

1/4 cup walnuts

1/2 teaspoon vanilla extract

1/4 teaspoon nutmeg

1 cup almond milk

Instructions:

1. Blend carrots, pineapple, and walnuts until creamy.

2. Add vanilla extract, nutmeg, and almond milk; blend again.

3. Pour into a glass and savor the carrot cake-inspired delight.

Tips for Crafting Kidney-Friendly Smoothies

Portion Control: Keep portion sizes in check to manage nutrient intake.

Liquid Base: Use hydrating bases like water, coconut water, or herbal teas to maintain fluid balance.

Personalization: Adjust recipes to individual preferences and dietary needs.

Experiment with Ingredients: Explore different combinations to find the flavors that suit your taste buds.

Limit High-Potassium Ingredients: Be mindful of the potassium content, especially in fruits like bananas and oranges.

Consult Healthcare Professionals: Seek advice from healthcare professionals or a registered dietitian for personalized guidance.

With these 15 delightful and kidney-friendly smoothie recipes, you can embark on a flavorful journey that supports your renal health. Always consult with healthcare professionals or a registered dietitian for personalized dietary advice based on individual health condition

Incorporating Smoothies into Daily Routine

Incorporating kidney-friendly smoothies into your daily routine is a delightful and handy strategy to improve renal function. Start your day with a colorful berry combination, or get a lunchtime pick-me-up with a tropical twist. Smoothies are a convenient way to incorporate critical nutrients, water, and antioxidant-rich foods into your diet. They are easily adjustable to specific taste preferences and provide a pleasant alternative to less kidney-friendly food. Making smoothies a regular part of your routine not only improves your nutritional intake but also establishes a pleasant habit that contributes to your overall well-being. Remember to speak with healthcare specialists for specialized recommendations based on your specific health needs.

Breakfast smoothie ideas

Breakfast smoothies are a delicious and nutritious way to start your day while addressing renal health. Incorporating kidney-friendly ingredients assures a balance of key nutrients without sacrificing flavor. Here's a thorough guide to making nourishing breakfast smoothies:

1. Berry Bliss Blast

Ingredients:

1/2 cup blueberries (fresh or frozen)

1/2 cup strawberries (fresh or frozen)

1/4 cup raspberries (fresh or frozen)

1/2 banana (fresh or frozen, peeled and sliced)

1 tablespoon chia seeds

1 cup water or coconut water

Instructions:

Blend all berries with chia seeds until smooth.

Adjust consistency with water or coconut water.

2. Tropical Sunrise Splash

Ingredients:

1/2 cup pineapple (fresh or frozen)

1/2 cup mango (fresh or frozen, peeled and diced)

1/4 cup cucumber (peeled and sliced)

1 tablespoon flaxseeds

1/2 teaspoon turmeric

1 cup coconut water

Instructions:

Blend pineapple, mango, and cucumber until smooth.

Add flaxseeds, turmeric, and coconut water; blend again.

3. Green Protein Powerhouse

Ingredients:

1 cup spinach (fresh or frozen)

1/2 cup kale (fresh or frozen)

1/2 banana (fresh or frozen, peeled and sliced)

1 tablespoon chia seeds

1/4 cup Greek yogurt

1 cup water or almond milk

Instructions:

Blend spinach, kale, and banana until smooth.

Add chia seeds, Greek yogurt, and water or almond milk; blend again.

4. Citrus Energy Elixir

Ingredients:

1/2 orange (peeled and segmented)

1/2 grapefruit (peeled and segmented)

1/2 cup cucumber (peeled and sliced)

1 tablespoon chia seeds

1/4 teaspoon ginger (freshly grated)

1 cup water or herbal tea

Instructions:

Blend orange, grapefruit, and cucumber until smooth.

Add chia seeds, ginger, and water or herbal tea; blend again.

5. Creamy Avocado Delight

Ingredients:

1/2 avocado

1/2 cup mixed berries (blueberries, raspberries, strawberries)

1 tablespoon flaxseeds

1/4 cup almond milk

1/4 cup water

Ice cubes (optional)

Instructions:

Combine all ingredients in a blender.

Blend until smooth and creamy.

If you want your smoothie to be colder, add ice cubes.

6. Peachy Oatmeal Dream

Ingredients:

1 cup peaches (fresh or frozen, peeled and sliced)

1/4 cup oats (uncooked)

1/2 teaspoon cinnamon

1/4 cup Greek yogurt

1 tablespoon chia seeds

1 cup almond milk

Instructions:

Blend peaches, oats, and cinnamon until smooth.

Add Greek yogurt, chia seeds, and almond milk; blend again.

7. Banana Walnut Wonder

Ingredients:

1/2 banana (fresh or frozen, peeled and sliced)

1/4 cup walnuts

1/4 cup oats (uncooked)

1/2 teaspoon vanilla extract

1/4 teaspoon cinnamon

1 cup almond milk

Instructions:

Blend banana, walnuts, oats, vanilla extract, and cinnamon until creamy.

Add almond milk; blend again.

8. Minty Melon Cooler

Ingredients:

1 cup cantaloupe (fresh or frozen, diced)

1/2 cup honeydew (fresh or frozen, diced)

1/4 cup mint leaves

1 tablespoon chia seeds

1/4 cup coconut water

1/4 cup water

Instructions:

Blend cantaloupe, honeydew, and mint leaves until smooth.

Add chia seeds, coconut water, and water; blend again.

9. Strawberry Basil Breeze

Ingredients:

1 cup strawberries (fresh or frozen)

1/4 cup basil leaves

1/2 cucumber (peeled and sliced)

1 tablespoon chia seeds

1/4 teaspoon ginger (freshly grated)

1 cup water or herbal tea

Instructions:

Blend strawberries, basil, and cucumber until smooth.

Add chia seeds, ginger, and water or herbal tea; blend again.

10. Coconut Berry Crush

Ingredients:

1/2 cup mixed berries (blueberries, raspberries, strawberries)

1/4 cup shredded coconut (unsweetened)

1/2 banana (fresh or frozen, peeled and sliced)

1 tablespoon chia seeds

1/4 cup coconut milk

1 cup water

Instructions:

1. Blend mixed berries, shredded coconut, and banana until smooth.

2. Add chia seeds, coconut milk, and water; blend again.

11. Cherry Almond Indulgence

Ingredients:

1/2 cup cherries (fresh or frozen, pitted)

1/4 cup almonds (unsalted)

1/2 cup cucumber (peeled and sliced)

1 tablespoon flaxseeds

1/4 teaspoon cinnamon

1 cup almond milk

Instructions:

1. Blend cherries, almonds, and cucumber until creamy.

2. Add flaxseeds, cinnamon, and almond milk; blend again.

12. Apple Pie Pleaser

Ingredients:

1 cup apples (peeled, cored, and diced)

1/2 teaspoon cinnamon

1/4 cup oats (uncooked)

1/2 cup Greek yogurt

1 tablespoon chia seeds

1 cup water or almond milk

Instructions:

1. Blend apples and cinnamon until smooth.

2. Add oats, Greek yogurt, chia seeds, and water or almond milk; blend again.

13. Blackberry Basil Fusion

Ingredients:

- 1/2 cup blackberries (fresh or frozen)

- 1/4 cup basil leaves

- 1/2 cup cucumber (peeled and sliced)

- 1 tablespoon chia seeds

- 1/4 cup coconut water

- 1/4 cup water

Instructions:

1. Blend blackberries, basil, and cucumber until smooth.

2. Add chia seeds, coconut water, and water; blend again.

14. Blueberry Lemon Zest

Ingredients:

1/2 cup blueberries (fresh or frozen)

Zest of 1 lemon

1/2 cup cucumber (peeled and sliced)

1 tablespoon chia seeds

1/4 cup Greek yogurt

1 cup water or coconut water

Instructions:

1. Blend blueberries, lemon zest, and cucumber until smooth.

2. Add chia seeds, Greek yogurt, and water or coconut water; blend again.

15. Carrot Cake Celebration

Ingredients:

1/2 cup carrots (peeled and sliced)

1/4 cup pineapple (fresh or frozen)

1/4 cup walnuts

1/2 teaspoon vanilla extract

1/4 teaspoon nutmeg

1 cup almond milk

Instructions:

1. Blend carrots, pineapple, and walnuts until creamy.

2. Add vanilla extract, nutmeg, and almond milk; blend again.

Tips for Crafting Kidney-Friendly Breakfast Smoothies:

Balance Nutrients: Include a mix of fruits, vegetables, protein, and healthy fats.

Control Portion Sizes: Be mindful of portion sizes to manage nutrient intake.

Hydrate Smartly: Use water, coconut water, or herbal teas as a base to maintain fluid balance.

Experiment with Add-Ins: Try adding ingredients like chia seeds, flaxseeds, or Greek yogurt for added texture and nutrition.

Personalize to Taste: Adjust recipes based on personal preferences and dietary needs.

Consult Healthcare Professionals: Seek guidance from healthcare professionals or a registered dietitian for personalized advice tailored to your specific health conditions.

Start your mornings on a vibrant note with these kidney-friendly breakfast smoothie ideas. By incorporating nutrient-dense and delicious ingredients, you can foster a healthy routine that supports your overall well-being. Always consult with healthcare professionals for personalized dietary advice based on individual health conditions.

Snacking can be both delightful and health-conscious with the incorporation of kidney-friendly smoothies. These options not only satisfy your taste buds but also provide essential nutrients, keeping renal health in mind. Here's a comprehensive guide to snack-time smoothie options:

1. Creamy Banana Almond Bliss

Ingredients:

1/2 banana (fresh or frozen, peeled and sliced)

1/4 cup almonds (unsalted)

1/4 cup Greek yogurt

1 tablespoon chia seeds

1/2 cup water or almond milk

Instructions:

Blend banana, almonds, and Greek yogurt until creamy.

Add chia seeds and water or almond milk; blend again.

2. Refreshing Cucumber Mint Cooler:

Ingredients:

1/2 cucumber (peeled and sliced)

1/4 cup mint leaves

1/2 cup green grapes

1 tablespoon chia seeds

1/4 teaspoon ginger (freshly grated)

1/2 cup water or coconut water

Instructions:

Blend cucumber, mint, and grapes until smooth.

Add chia seeds, ginger, and water or coconut water; blend again.

3. Berries and Oats Marvel

Ingredients:

1/2 cup mixed berries (blueberries, raspberries, strawberries)

1/4 cup oats (uncooked)

1/4 cup Greek yogurt

1 tablespoon flaxseeds

1/2 cup water or almond milk

Instructions:

Blend mixed berries and oats until smooth.

Add Greek yogurt, flaxseeds, and water or almond milk; blend again.

4. Pineapple Coconut Delight

Ingredients:

1/2 cup pineapple (fresh or frozen)

1/4 cup shredded coconut (unsweetened)

1/2 banana (fresh or frozen, peeled and sliced)

1 tablespoon chia seeds

1/2 cup coconut water

Instructions:

Blend pineapple, shredded coconut, and banana until smooth.

Add the chia seeds and coconut water and mix again.

5. Cherry Vanilla Symphony:

Ingredients:

1/2 cup cherries (fresh or frozen, pitted)

1/2 teaspoon vanilla extract

1/4 cup almonds (unsalted)

1 tablespoon flaxseeds

1/2 cup water or almond milk

Instructions:

Blend cherries and vanilla extract until smooth.

Add almonds, flaxseeds, and water or almond milk; blend again.

6. Kiwi Lime Zinger

Ingredients:

2 kiwis (peeled and sliced)

Zest and juice of 1 lime

1/2 cup green grapes

1 tablespoon chia seeds

1/2 cup water or coconut water

Instructions:

Blend kiwis, lime zest, and lime juice until smooth.

Add green grapes, chia seeds, and water or coconut water; blend again.

7. Spinach Apple Elegance

Ingredients:

1 cup spinach (fresh or frozen)

1/2 cup apples (peeled, cored, and diced)

1/4 cup Greek yogurt

1 tablespoon chia seeds

1/2 cup water or almond milk

Instructions:

Blend spinach and apples until smooth.

Add Greek yogurt, chia seeds, and water or almond milk; blend again.

8. Mango Ginger Infusion

Ingredients:

1 cup mango (fresh or frozen, peeled and diced)

1/4 teaspoon ginger (freshly grated)

1/4 cup cashews (unsalted)

1 tablespoon flaxseeds

1/2 cup water or coconut water

Instructions:

Blend mango and ginger until creamy.

Add cashews, flaxseeds, and water or coconut water; blend again.

9. Blueberry Basil Bliss

Ingredients:

1/2 cup blueberries (fresh or frozen)

1/4 cup basil leaves

1/4 cup cucumber (peeled and sliced)

1 tablespoon chia seeds

1/2 cup water or coconut water

Instructions:

Blend blueberries, basil, and cucumber until smooth.

Add chia seeds and water or coconut water; blend again.

10. Pear Honey Harmony

Ingredients:

1/2 pear (peeled and diced)

1 tablespoon honey

1/4 cup almonds (unsalted)

1 tablespoon chia seeds

1/2 cup water or almond milk

Instructions:

1. Blend pear and honey until smooth.

2. Add almonds, chia seeds, and water or almond milk; blend again.

Tips for Crafting Kidney-Friendly Snack-Time Smoothies

Moderate Portions: Control portion sizes to manage nutrient intake.

Mindful Ingredients: Opt for kidney-friendly options, avoiding high-potassium fruits and excessive dairy.

Hydration Balance: Incorporate hydrating bases like water, coconut water, or herbal teas.

Protein Boost: Include sources of protein such as Greek yogurt, nuts, or seeds.

Experiment with Flavors: Explore diverse flavor combinations to keep your snacks exciting.

Personalize to Preferences: Adjust recipes based on taste preferences and dietary needs.

Consult Healthcare Professionals: Seek guidance from healthcare professionals or a registered dietitian for personalized advice tailored to your specific health conditions.

By choosing kidney-friendly ingredients and being mindful of nutritional balance, these snack-time smoothie options provide a tasty and nutritious way to indulge between meals. Always consult with healthcare professionals for personalized dietary advice based on individual health conditions.

Preparing smoothies for hydration

Staying hydrated is essential for good health, and including hydrating smoothies in your daily routine can be a tasty and fun approach to satisfy your fluid requirements. Here's a thorough approach to producing smoothies aimed at improving hydration

Importance of Hydration in Smoothies

Hydration is essential for a variety of bodily activities, including fluid balance, digestion, and temperature regulation. Smoothies can help you stay hydrated by integrating water-rich ingredients that also include vitamins and minerals.

Hydrating Ingredients: Base Liquids.

Water is the ultimate hydrator, keeping you rejuvenated.

Coconut water contains electrolytes for enhanced hydration.

Herbal teas provide flavor while also hydrating.

High-water-content fruits

Watermelon: Made up primarily of water and high in vitamins.

Cucumber is a hydrating vegetable that combines well in smoothies.

Strawberries: Juicy and tasty, with a moisturizing effect.

Leafy Greens

Spinach is hydrating and nutrient-dense without compromising flavor.

Cabbage provides hydration and a little sweetness to smoothies.

Hydration-Boosting Smoothie Recipes

Watermelon Mint Refresher:

Ingredients:

2 cups fresh watermelon (seedless, cubed)

1/4 cup mint leaves

1 cup coconut water

Ice cubes (optional)

Instructions:

Blend watermelon and mint until smooth.

Add coconut water and ice cubes; blend again.

Cooling Cucumber Citrus Splash

Ingredients:

1 cucumber (peeled and sliced)

Juice of 2 limes

1 cup green grapes

1/2 cup water

Fresh basil leaves (optional)

Instructions:

Blend cucumber, lime juice, and grapes until smooth.

Add water and basil leaves; blend again.

Berry Hydration Boost

Ingredients:

1 cup mixed berries (blueberries, raspberries, strawberries)

1/2 cup coconut water

1/2 cup water

1 tablespoon chia seeds

Instructions:

Blend mixed berries with coconut water.

Add water and chia seeds; blend again.

Tips for Optimal Hydration:

Include Electrolyte-Rich Ingredients:

Add ingredients like coconut water or electrolyte-infused beverages to support hydration.

Experiment with Hydrating Greens.

Incorporate hydrating greens like celery or lettuce for a nutrient boost.

Use Frozen Fruits.

Frozen fruits not only add a refreshing chill but also contribute to overall fluid intake.

Monitor Sugar Content:

Be mindful of added sugars, as excessive sugar intake can contribute to dehydration.

Prefer Whole Fruits:

Opt for whole fruits in smoothies to retain fiber, aiding in hydration.

Hydrating Add-Ins:

Consider adding aloe vera juice or coconut water ice cubes for extra hydration.

Smoothies designed for hydration are a delightful and effective method to meet your daily fluid requirements. You may make refreshing mixes that promote general well-being by using water-rich components and hydrated bases. Remember to tailor recipes to your taste preferences and get specialized guidance from healthcare professionals, especially if you have a specific health problem.

CHAPTER FOUR

LIFESTYLE AND RENAL HEALTH

Lifestyle decisions have a significant impact on kidney health. Maintaining a balanced diet with low sodium intake, staying hydrated, and managing weight through regular exercise are all essential for kidney health. Blood pressure control, smoking cessation, and moderation of alcohol consumption all reduce the chance of developing renal disease. Effective management of chronic illnesses such as diabetes improves overall kidney health. Stress reduction techniques and frequent health check-ups also help kidney function. Adherence to recommended drugs and a holistic approach to a kidney-friendly lifestyle are essential. Individuals should seek specialized guidance from healthcare professionals, with recommendations tailored to their specific health conditions.

Exercise and Physical Activity

Physical activity is an essential component of general well-being, with far-reaching health benefits, including a positive impact on renal health. This section evaluates the benefits, considerations, and techniques involved with exercise and physical activity, focusing on their involvement in renal health.

The Interconnectedness of Exercise and Renal Health

Cardiovascular Health and Circulation

Regular exercise is essential for maintaining cardiovascular health and improving blood circulation. This is especially important for renal health because the kidneys rely on a steady blood flow to carry out their essential tasks. Improved blood flow ensures that the kidneys receive appropriate oxygen and nutrients, allowing them to work optimally.

Weight Management and Renal Wellness

Weight control is inextricably tied to kidney health. Obesity is a substantial risk factor for kidney disease, and exercise can help you lose or maintain weight. Physical activity burns calories, builds lean muscle mass, and regulates metabolism, all of which help you reach and maintain a healthy weight.

Physical activity helps control blood pressure.

Hypertension (high blood pressure) is a primary cause of renal damage. Regular exercise has been demonstrated to lower blood pressure, which reduces the risk of renal issues. The mechanisms include blood vessel dilatation and better cardiovascular function.

Exercise's Effect on Insulin Sensitivity and Diabetes Management

Regular physical exercise improves insulin sensitivity, which is crucial for diabetes management. Diabetes is a major risk factor for kidney disease, and exercise can help reduce that risk by improving glucose management. Controlling blood sugar levels with physical activity improves both diabetes control and kidney health.

Muscle and bone health in the context of kidney function.

Strength training and other weight-bearing workouts help to maintain bone density and muscle strength. While the direct relationship between muscle and bone health and kidney function is not often clear, overall physical resilience is critical, particularly for people with chronic renal disease.

Reducing Inflammation and Stress via Exercise

Chronic inflammation is linked to a variety of health conditions, including kidney troubles. Regular exercise contains anti-inflammatory properties, which may reduce the incidence of inflammation-related kidney disorders. Furthermore, exercise is a proven stress reliever, which indirectly benefits kidney health by lowering the risk of stress-related illnesses.

Quality Sleep and Its Relationship to Exercise

Exercise has been shown to improve sleep quality, and getting enough sleep is important for overall health, including kidney function. The association between sleep and exercise is bidirectional, with regular physical activity helping to improve sleep patterns.

Fluid Regulation: Sweating and Hydration.

Physical activity causes sweating, which helps to eliminate toxins from the body. Proper hydration during exercise is essential to avoid dehydration and maintain renal function. Adequate fluid consumption helps to maintain electrolyte balance and allows the kidneys to effectively filter waste materials.

Considerations for Kidney Health in Exercise.

While exercise is typically excellent for renal health, individuals with kidney difficulties should approach physical activity with the following considerations:

Individualized Approach.

Exercise plans should be adjusted to each person's specific health situation. Fluid intake, activity type and intensity, and potential kidney strain should all be carefully examined. Individuals with kidney issues should speak with a healthcare provider or a renal dietician to develop a specific workout regimen.

Types of Exercise and their Roles

Different types of exercises provide varying benefits:

Aerobic exercise.

Walking, running, cycling, and swimming all promote cardiovascular health, which indirectly benefits renal function by ensuring a consistent blood supply to the kidney.

Strength Training

Building muscle strength through resistance training improves overall physical fitness. While direct links between muscle strength and renal function may not be obvious, strength training's overall advantages promote an active and healthy lifestyle.

Flexibility and Balance Training

Yoga and tai chi improve flexibility and balance. While not directly affecting kidney function, these activities improve general physical well-being and can be included in a comprehensive exercise regimen.

Hydration and Exercise

Proper hydration is essential during exercise to avoid dehydration, especially for people who have kidney difficulties. Maintaining a balance between fluid intake and output is critical. It is best to speak with a healthcare expert to establish your individual hydration needs.

Frequency and Duration of Exercise

Consistent physical activity is essential for general health benefits. While guidelines for exercise frequency and duration vary, frequent, moderate-intensity exercise is typically recommended. Individual needs must be considered, and it is critical to heed the body's messages.

Medical Guidelines for Exercise

Individuals with pre-existing health ailments, such as kidney problems, should consult a doctor before beginning an exercise program. Healthcare specialists can make individualized suggestions depending on an individual's health situation, ensuring that the fitness regimen they choose is appropriate for their overall well-being.

Exercise and physical exercise are essential for maintaining kidney health. The benefits are numerous, ranging from cardiovascular health to weight management, blood pressure control, and indirect impacts to stress reduction and better sleep. However, a one-size-fits-all strategy is not appropriate, especially for people who have kidney issues. A tailored, cautious, and well-informed strategy, guided by healthcare specialists, ensures that exercise becomes an important part of overall renal health. Adopting a balanced and personalized exercise plan benefits not just renal function but also the overall health of the individual.

Benefits of regular exercise for renal health

Regular exercise is not only essential for overall well-being, but it also has a significant impact on the health of important organs such as the kidneys. This extensive review digs into the numerous benefits of regular exercise for renal health, highlighting the interconnection between physical activity and the proper functioning of these essential organs.

1. Regular exercise promotes cardiovascular health and efficient blood circulation. The heart delivers blood to every region of the body, including the kidneys. Improved

cardiovascular performance ensures that the kidneys receive adequate blood flow, allowing for efficient waste filtering and supporting their critical tasks.

2. Exercise helps regulate blood pressure and manage hypertension, which is important for kidney health. Hypertension (high blood pressure) is a primary cause of renal damage. Regular physical activity helps to treat and prevent hypertension by improving blood vessel flexibility and lowering overall resistance.

3. Exercise helps manage diabetes and improve insulin sensitivity, reducing the risk of kidney damage. Regular physical activity improves insulin sensitivity and glucose management. Exercise improves overall renal health by regulating blood sugar levels and lowering the incidence of diabetes-related kidney problems.

4. Weight Management and Obesity Prevention: Keeping a healthy weight is essential for kidney health, and exercise is a vital factor in weight management. Obesity is strongly connected to the onset and progression of renal disease.

Regular physical exercise burns calories, increases lean muscle mass, and regulates metabolism, all of which serve to prevent and control obesity.

5. Reduced Inflammation with Anti-Inflammatory Effects: Chronic inflammation is a risk factor for kidney disease. Regular exercise provides significant anti-inflammatory benefits, which may reduce the incidence of inflammation-related kidney disorders. This anti-inflammatory effect extends beyond the kidneys, benefiting general health.

6. Exercise can lower stress and improve mental well-being. Stress management is crucial for general health, including renal function. Lower stress levels improve the body's ability to maintain a healthy balance and promote kidney health. Exercise's mood-enhancing benefits help to increase mental well-being, which in turn helps physiological equilibrium.

7. Improved Sleep Quality and Restorative Benefits: Regular exercise promotes better sleep patterns and quality. Adequate, restorative sleep is essential for general health,

and the benefits extend to kidney function. Quality sleep promotes the body's optimal performance, assisting the kidneys in their critical duties.

Weight-bearing exercises, such as strength training, can improve muscle and bone strength, leading to increased physical resilience. Overall physical resilience is critical for those managing chronic renal disease because it helps prevent musculoskeletal disorders and promotes overall well-being.

9. Sweating and Hydration: Physical exercise promotes sweating, which helps eliminate toxins from the body. Proper hydration during exercise is critical for preventing dehydration and maintaining renal function. Maintaining a balance between fluid intake and output is critical, and those with renal problems should speak with a doctor about tailored hydration guidelines.

10. Better Mental Health and Mood Enhancement:

Regular exercise improves mood and has a good impact on mental health. Exercise is linked to greater mood and fewer symptoms of despair and anxiety. Positive mental health indirectly promotes overall physiological equilibrium, including kidney health.

11. Regular physical activity can strengthen the immune system and improve overall well-being. While not directly related to renal health, a strong immune system promotes overall well-being by helping to prevent infections and illnesses that might harm the kidneys.

12. Social Engagement and Community Benefits: Group activities and sports promote social bonds. Social involvement is an important part of overall well-being and may improve mental and emotional health. While not directly related to renal health, the communal benefits of exercise add to a more holistic approach to health.

13. Long-term Renal Health Advantages and Chronic Kidney Disease Prevention:

Regular exercise can help prevent the development and progression of chronic kidney disease by addressing a variety of risk factors such as high blood pressure, diabetes, and obesity. The cumulative effect of exercise on these risk variables provides a foundation for long-term renal health.

14. Individualized Exercise Plans and Adjusted Approaches: Exercise plans should be adjusted to an individual's health state, taking into account exercise type and intensity, pre-existing health issues, and preferences. A tailored approach guarantees that exercise complements an individual's general well-being and addresses specific health concerns.

Regular exercise appears as an effective tool for developing and sustaining kidney health. Its advantages extend across a wide range of physiological and psychological domains, from cardiovascular health and blood pressure control to diabetes treatment, weight regulation, and immune system support. Regular exercise, together with a balanced diet and other healthy habits, provides a comprehensive strategy for maintaining kidney health.

While the benefits are numerous, individuals, particularly those with preexisting health concerns, should exercise caution and seek advice from healthcare specialists. Consulting with medical professionals guarantees a specific, safe, and successful strategy for obtaining and maintaining renal health through regular physical exercise. Practicing a balanced and personalized exercise plan benefits not only kidney health but also the individual's overall health and longevity.

Suitable exercises for individuals with kidney issues

When dealing with kidney troubles, adding appropriate activities to one's regimen is critical for maintaining general well-being while protecting the health of these key organs. This comprehensive section evaluates a wide range of workouts that are widely regarded as safe and effective for people with kidney problems, emphasizing the significance of tailored approaches and regular consultation with healthcare professionals.

1. Low-impact aerobic exercises.

Walking: This low-impact activity is gentle on the joints and cardiovascular system, making it a good alternative for people who have kidney problems. Walking may be tailored to different fitness levels, making it a customized workout option.

Stationary cycling provides cardiovascular advantages without putting too much strain on the joints, making it an efficient technique to boost heart health and overall well-being.

2. Swimming and water aerobics.

Swimming: Because water's buoyancy lessens the joint impact, swimming is an excellent workout for people who have kidney problems. It delivers a full-body workout and is beneficial to cardiovascular health.

Water Aerobics: Combining aerobic workouts with the buoyancy of water, water aerobics is a low-impact way to increase strength and flexibility.

3. Yoga and Tai Chi

Yoga, known for its emphasis on gentle movements, flexibility, and relaxation, can be tailored to suit a variety of fitness levels. Certain poses and sequences improve flexibility, balance, and stress reduction.

Tai Chi is characterized by slow, controlled motions that improve balance and flexibility. It is ideal for anyone with varying fitness levels and is especially mild on the joints.

4. Strength Training With Light Weights

Light Dumbbells: Adding light weights to strength training routine helps maintain muscle strength without putting undue strain on the body. To avoid strain on the kidneys, aim for higher repetitions with lesser weights.

Resistance Bands: These bands provide resistance for strength training without the use of heavy weights, making them a versatile and safe solution for people with renal concerns.

5. Flexibility exercises.

Stretching Routines: Gentle stretching exercises increase flexibility and lower the chance of muscle tightness. Flexibility is vital for overall joint health, and it might be especially useful for people with kidney concerns.

Range of Motion Exercises: These exercises aim to preserve joint mobility without putting undue strain on the body, hence improving general physical well-being.

6. Breathing exercises and relaxation techniques.

Deep breathing exercises improve relaxation and can be easily incorporated into any training regimen. It helps to reduce stress and promote mental well-being.

Meditation Practices: Meditation, which focuses on mindfulness and calming the mind, helps to reduce stress and improves general mental and emotional health.

7. Seated exercises

Chair Aerobics: Adapted aerobic workouts conducted while seated, designed specifically for people with restricted mobility. This alternative provides low-impact training, making it appropriate for people with renal concerns.

Seated Yoga: Modified yoga poses that may be performed while sitting offer the benefits of traditional yoga while appealing to people of varying fitness levels.

8. Cardiovascular exercises with monitoring.

Elliptical Trainer: The elliptical trainer provides a low-impact yet effective cardiovascular workout that is easy on the joints. Individuals should keep track of their intensity and duration, and adjust as needed based on their fitness level and comfort.

Treadmill with Handrails: Walking on a treadmill with handrails provides more stability and control, making it an appropriate alternative for people who have renal problems. Take care not to overexert yourself.

9. Guided Exercise Classes

Physical Therapy Programs: Physical therapists lead tailored exercise programs that give an organized and personalized approach to those with renal difficulties. These programs emphasize rehabilitation and total physical well-being.

Renal-Specific Exercise Sessions: Some fitness instructors specialize in creating exercise sessions with a thorough awareness of kidney health concerns. Participating in such sessions ensures that the fitness routine meets the specific demands of those with kidney problems.

10. Hydration and Regular Monitoring.

Proper Hydration: Staying hydrated is critical for people with kidney problems. Proper fluid consumption promotes electrolyte balance and renal function. Hydration is particularly important during activity.

Regular Monitoring: People with renal problems should pay close attention to how their bodies react to exercise. Monitoring for any unwanted effects or pain is critical, and changes to the workout plan may be required based on individual responses.

11. Individualized Exercise Plans

Consultation with Healthcare Professionals: Before beginning any fitness routine, people with kidney problems should visit their healthcare team, which includes nephrologists, physical therapists, and renal dietitians. These pros can offer valuable insights into creating tailored fitness routines.

Exercise regimens should be adjusted to each individual's health state, taking into account aspects such as exercise kind and intensity, pre-existing health issues, and personal preferences. A personalized method guarantees that the workout program is consistent with an individual's general well-being.

12. Use caution when performing heavy lifting.

Avoiding Heavy Weightlifting: Although strength training is important, heavy lifting can put a strain on the kidneys. To reap the benefits of strength training without putting undue strain on the kidneys, use light weights and increase the number of repetitions.

13. Consistent and Gradual Progression

Consistent Exercise Routine: Regular, moderate-intensity exercise is frequently more beneficial than occasional intensive workouts. Establishing a steady practice improves overall health and helps people with renal problems maintain their fitness levels.

Gradual Progression: As fitness improves, people can progressively increase the intensity and duration of their workouts. This slow approach enables the body to adapt while reducing the risk of overexertion.

14. Regular Health Check-Ups

Monitoring Kidney Function: People with kidney problems should see their doctor regularly. These examinations include assessments of kidney function and overall health, allowing healthcare experts to make informed suggestions and changes to exercise regimens.

Adjusting Exercise regimens Based on Health Status: Healthcare providers might modify exercise regimens based on an individual's overall health. This involves adjusting the workout plan to reflect changes in kidney function or addressing any new health concerns.

Exercises appropriate for people with renal problems should be varied, adaptive, and adapted to each individual's specific needs. The basic aim is to promote overall health while reducing kidney stress. Combining low-impact aerobic activities, flexibility routines, strength training with light weights, and relaxation techniques results in a well-rounded approach to physical activity. Regular interaction with healthcare professionals ensures that the chosen activities are appropriate for an individual's health situation, contributing to the overall management of kidney health.

Monitoring Kidney Function: People with kidney problems should see their doctor regularly. These examinations include assessments of kidney function and overall health, allowing healthcare experts to make informed suggestions and changes to exercise regimens.

Adjusting Exercise regimens Based on Health Status: Healthcare providers might modify exercise regimens based on an individual's overall health. This involves adjusting the workout plan to reflect changes in kidney function or addressing any new health concerns.

Exercises appropriate for people with renal problems should be varied, adaptive, and adapted to each individual's specific needs. The basic aim is to promote overall health while reducing kidney stress. Combining low-impact aerobic activities, flexibility routines, strength training with light weights, and relaxation techniques results in a well-rounded approach to physical activity. Regular interaction with healthcare professionals ensures that the chosen activities are appropriate for an individual's health situation, contributing to the overall management of kidney health.

Hydration and its Role

Hydration is essential for overall health, especially kidney function. Adequate water consumption is required for proper kidney function, which aids in the elimination of waste products and toxins from the body. Proper hydration helps manage electrolyte balance, blood pressure, and fluid levels, which aids in the prevention of kidney stones and urinary tract infections. Maintaining an optimal fluid balance is especially important for people with renal problems. Finding a balance between hydration and kidney health requires unique considerations, and engaging with healthcare specialists ensures that fluid consumption is tailored to an individual's specific needs, encouraging optimal kidney function and general well-being.

Proper hydration is an essential component of general health and well-being, influencing many physiological systems throughout the body. This in-depth review digs into the multiple importance of remaining hydrated, highlighting its role in organ function, electrolyte balance, blood pressure regulation, temperature control, joint health, cognitive function, digestive well-being, and more.

1. Optimal Organ Function

Renal Health: The kidneys, which filter waste products and poisons from the blood, rely on enough hydration. Adequate fluid consumption allows the kidneys to effectively discharge these chemicals through urine, promoting normal renal function.

2. Electrolyte Balance.

Sodium, Potassium, and Electrolytes: Hydration is inextricably related to maintaining an equilibrium of important electrolytes like sodium and potassium. These electrolytes are essential for neuron activity, muscular contractions, and maintaining fluid balance within and outside cells.

3. Blood Pressure Regulation

Fluid Volume and Blood Pressure: Hydration helps regulate blood volume, which affects blood pressure. Maintaining correct fluid levels aids in blood pressure regulation, lowering the risk of hypertension and other cardiovascular problems.

4. Temperature Regulation.

Sweating and the Cooling Mechanism: Hydration is required for the body's cooling mechanism to function properly. Adequate fluid balance avoids dehydration and ensures proper temperature control during physical activity and exposure to hot weather.

5. Joint Lubrication and Mobility

Hydration promotes the development of synovial fluid, a lubricant found in joints. Well-lubricated joints improve mobility, minimize friction, and promote overall joint health.

6. Digestive Health

Proper water supports the development of digestive enzymes and saliva. This helps with the digestive process, from breaking down food in the mouth to improving nutrient absorption in the digestive tract.

7. Cognitive Function

Dehydration can negatively affect cognitive function, causing difficulties with concentration, attention, and memory. Maintaining sufficient hydration promotes optimal blood flow to the brain, which improves cognitive ability.

8. Cellular Processes

Hydration facilitates nutrient transport and waste elimination. This is crucial for cellular functions, energy production, and general tissue and organ health.

9. Skin Health Moisture Retention

Proper hydration improves skin elasticity, moisture retention, and overall health. Dehydration can cause dry skin, accelerated aging, and increased susceptibility to skin conditions.

10. Urinary Tract Health.

Prevention of Infections: Proper hydration helps to eliminate bacteria from the urinary tract, lowering the risk of infections. This is very important for the health of the urinary system.

11. Improved Exercise Performance and Recovery

Proper hydration is essential for athletes and active people. Maintaining correct fluid balance increases endurance, helps regulate temperature during activity, and promotes good post-exercise recovery.

12. Weight Management Appetite Regulation

Proper hydration can impact appetite regulation. The body might mistake thirst for hunger, resulting in excessive calorie consumption. Staying hydrated may assist prevent overeating.

13. Detoxification Processes

Toxin Elimination: Hydration helps the body's natural detoxification process. Proper fluid intake aids in the removal of metabolic wastes and environmental pollutants via urine and sweat.

14. Individual Hydration Needs

Age, Activity Levels, and Health Status: Recognizing that hydration requirements vary depending on age, activity level, climate, and health state is critical. Individualized hydration regimens ensure that fluid consumption is in line with unique demands.

15. Hydration and Aging Considerations

Individuals' sensation of thirst may weaken as they age, making it critical to stay hydrated on purpose. Proper fluid consumption promotes organ function, joint health, and cognitive well-being in the elderly population.

Proper hydration is essential for more than just quenching one's thirst. It is intricately woven into the fabric of overall health, impacting organ function, maintaining electrolyte balance, regulating blood pressure, promoting temperature management, improving joint health, and maintaining cognitive function. Recognizing the connection of hydration to many physiological systems emphasizes its critical role in fostering health and vigor.

Individuals are advised to develop mindful water consumption habits, acknowledging that hydration requirements vary and can be influenced by age, activity level, and health status.

Choosing the right beverages for kidney health

Ensuring kidney health requires a comprehensive approach that goes beyond dietary considerations and includes the beverages we consume. The fluids we consume are critical to maintaining normal kidney function, fluid balance, and overall well-being. This comprehensive guide examines the significance of choosing the proper beverages for kidney health, including insights into ideal selections, moderation, and beverages to limit or avoid.

1. Hydration and Kidney Health.

Water as the cornerstone: Adequate hydration is essential for kidney function. Water is the foundation of fluid intake, delivering necessary hydration without adding calories, sweets, or additions. It is the purest and most natural way to enhance kidney function by encouraging waste clearance via urine.

2. Herbal teas and infusions.

Natural, calorie-free options: Herbal teas and infusions provide a tasty alternative to plain water. Chamomile, mint, and hibiscus are examples of varieties that not only help with hydration but may also provide health advantages. Importantly, they are caffeine-free, making them ideal for people looking to restrict their caffeine intake.

3. Consume fresh fruit juices in moderation.

Nutrient-Rich Options: While fresh fruit juices can provide critical vitamins and minerals, they should be consumed in moderation. Choose natural fruit juices with no added sugars to guarantee that the nutritional benefits are not overshadowed by an excessive sugar intake. Limiting portion sizes is critical for managing sugar consumption.

4. Nutrient-dense and Low in Sodium

Vegetable juices, especially those with low sodium content, provide a nutrient-dense hydration option. These beverages contain critical vitamins and antioxidants without the high sugar content commonly associated with fruit juices.

5. Coconut Water

A natural source of electrolytes, including potassium. It is a refreshing choice, especially after light physical exertion, and helps replace both fluids and electrolytes.

6. Limiting caffeinated and sugary beverages.

Caffeine and Diuretic Effects: While moderate caffeine use is normally tolerated, excessive intake may result in increased urine output. Caffeine is present in coffee, tea, and some drinks. Caffeine use should be limited for patients with kidney problems since excessive diuresis can disrupt fluid balance.

7. Alcohol in Moderation

Moderate alcohol consumption might lead to dehydration and stress on the kidneys. Moderation is recommended, and people with renal problems should contact their doctors about their alcohol consumption to make sure it fits into their overall health plan.

8. Limit Soda and Carbonated Drinks

Concerns about Phosphorus Content: Certain sodas and carbonated drinks may contain high quantities of phosphorus, which can be harmful to people who have renal problems. Managing phosphorus intake is critical for kidney health, and restricting the consumption of certain beverages can help achieve this objective.

9. Diluted fruit juices and infused water.

Reducing Sugar Intake: Diluting fruit juices with water or choosing infused water with natural flavors is a technique to improve taste without drastically increasing sugar intake. This allows people to enjoy flavored beverages while remaining careful of their sugar intake.

10. Avoiding Energy Drinks.

Energy drinks generally include high levels of caffeine and sugar, which can be harmful to kidney health. These beverages should be avoided or consumed in moderation, particularly by people with kidney issues.

11. Managing Sodium Intake

Reading Beverage Labels: Understanding the salt content in beverages, particularly bottled and canned drinks, is critical. High salt intake can cause fluid retention and raised blood pressure, affecting kidney function.

12. Selecting Low-Phosphorus Options.

Phosphorus and Kidney Health: Individuals with renal difficulties should limit their phosphorus consumption. Choosing low-phosphorus beverages helps to manage phosphorus levels and promotes kidney health. It is advisable to check labels for phosphorus content.

13. Healthcare Professionals' Individualized Recommendations

Each person's health is unique, therefore consulting with healthcare professionals such as nephrologists and nutritionists is crucial. These professionals can make tailored recommendations for fluid intake, taking into account specific dietary constraints and health concerns.

14. Water Intake and Physical Activity.

Adjusting for Exercise: Physical exercise can increase fluid requirements, particularly in cases of sweating. Adjusting water intake to compensate for fluid loss during exercise is critical for staying hydrated, improving kidney function, and increasing overall fitness.

15. Hydration Monitoring.

Listening to Body cues: Paying attention to your body's cues, such as thirst, is critical to staying hydrated. Thirst is a natural indication that the body requires fluids. Regularly monitoring hydration levels promotes a healthy fluid balance.

Our beverage choices have a significant impact on renal health. Optimal hydration is achieved by a balanced strategy that prioritizes water intake while taking other beverages in moderation. Herbal teas, vegetable juices, and coconut water are tasty options, while diluted fruit juices and infused water provide variety without sacrificing health. Being aware of the caffeine, sugar, alcohol, and sodium content of beverages, as well as seeking individualized guidance from healthcare specialists, allows people to make informed decisions that benefit kidney health. Individuals who incorporate these concerns into their daily lives can take proactive actions to maintain optimal kidney function and overall well-being.

Stress Management

In today's fast-paced and demanding world, good stress management is critical to sustaining mental and emotional health. Stress, if left ignored, can have serious consequences for physical and mental health. Implementing stress-management strategies is critical for developing resilience and leading a healthy life. Mindfulness, deep breathing techniques, and regular physical activity can all help alleviate stress. Creating healthy boundaries, prioritizing self-care, and getting help from friends, family, or professionals are all important aspects of stress management. Individuals who recognize and manage stressors proactively can create a resilient mentality, improve their general quality of life, and navigate life's problems more easily.

Impact of stress on renal health

Stress, an inescapable feature of modern life, has a significant impact on overall health, even affecting the precise functioning of the renal system. The kidneys, which are responsible for maintaining fluid and electrolyte balance, regulating blood pressure, and removing waste, are vulnerable to the effects of stress. This comprehensive review digs into the various ways in which stress can affect renal health, evaluating physiological reactions, potential repercussions, and techniques for reducing stress-related kidney damage.

1. Physiological Responses to Stress

Chronic stress triggers a series of physiological responses, principally activating the "fight or flight" response. This response involves the production of stress chemicals, including cortisol and adrenaline, which can have a significant impact on the entire body, including the kidneys.

Hormonal fluctuations

Chronic stress causes elevated cortisol levels, which can contribute to hormonal abnormalities. Cortisol, often known as the stress hormone, helps the body respond to stress by regulating metabolism, blood sugar, and immunological function. However, chronic exposure to elevated cortisol levels can disrupt these processes.

Blood pressure elevation

One of the immediate effects of stress is an increase in blood pressure. Stress causes the release of adrenaline, which constricts blood vessels and increases blood pressure. Chronic high blood pressure is especially bad for renal health because it puts the delicate blood vessels in the kidneys in danger.

2. Impact on Renal Blood Flow.

The kidneys are highly vascular organs that rely on adequate blood flow for proper function. Stress-induced sympathetic nervous system activation can result in vasoconstriction, which causes blood vessels to narrow. This vasoconstriction may impair renal blood flow, reducing the kidneys' ability to filter blood properly.

Reduced glomerular filtration rate (GFR).

The glomerular filtration rate (GFR) is an important indication of renal function since it represents the rate at which the kidneys filter blood. Chronic stress can cause prolonged vasoconstriction and high blood pressure, both of which can lead to a decrease in GFR. Reduced GFR indicates decreased filtration and removal of waste materials from circulation.

3. Inflammation and oxidative stress.

Chronic stress is strongly connected to an increase in inflammation throughout the body. Inflammation, a component of the immune system, is a double-edged sword. Acute inflammation is a protective mechanism, but prolonged inflammation can cause tissue damage. The kidneys, which are rich in blood arteries and fragile tissues, are prone to inflammation caused by stress.

Stress-induced inflammation can harm renal tissues, potentially causing kidney disease. Inflammatory mediators can alter the normal function of renal cells and structures, accelerating the evolution of renal diseases.

Oxidative Stress

Stress can also cause oxidative stress, which is defined by an imbalance in the generation of reactive oxygen species (ROS) and the body's ability to neutralize them. Oxidative stress can cause cellular damage, damaging renal cells and contributing to the onset or progression of kidney disease.

4. Exacerbation of Existing Kidney Conditions

Individuals with pre-existing kidney diseases, such as chronic kidney disease (CKD), may be more susceptible to the effects of stress. Chronic stress can hasten the advancement of preexisting renal diseases and raise the risk of complications.

Impact on Pre-Existing Conditions

Stress-induced physiological changes, such as raised blood pressure and inflammation, can exacerbate the damage that already exists in people with CKD. Effective stress management is critical to decreasing the progression of renal disease in this population.

Association with Kidney Stones

Stress has been linked to an increased chance of getting kidney stones. The complex interplay of stress hormones, mineral metabolism, and fluid balance may lead to the production of kidney stones.

5. Immune System Modulation.

Chronic stress affects the immune system, leaving people more vulnerable to illnesses. In terms of renal health, infections are a serious threat to the kidneys, potentially leading to complications such as kidney infections or glomerulonephritis.

Weakening Immune Response

Stress-induced immunosuppression can impair the body's defense against infections. Infections that reach the kidneys can cause inflammation and damage to renal tissues.

6. Behavioral Aspects and Lifestyle Choices

Stress frequently drives people to engage in coping techniques, which may involve unhealthy habits that influence renal health.

Unhealthy coping mechanisms

Common stress-related behaviors include smoking, excessive alcohol intake, and poor food choices. These activities can lead to hypertension, inflammation, and oxidative stress, all of which have a poor impact on kidney function.

Disrupted Sleep Patterns

Chronic stress can alter sleep patterns, resulting in insufficient or poor-quality sleep. Sleep difficulties have been related to poor overall health and may contribute to kidney disease.

7. Strategies for Reducing Stress-Related Renal Harm

Effective stress management is critical for maintaining renal health and preventing or minimizing stress-induced kidney damage.

Stress Management Techniques

Incorporating stress management practices into your daily routine can dramatically lessen the physiological impact of stress on the kidneys. Mindfulness, meditation, and deep breathing techniques are powerful ways to promote relaxation and reduce the body's stress reaction.

Regular exercise.

Regular physical activity is believed to lower stress and improve general well-being. Exercise improves blood pressure regulation and may have an indirect favorable effect on renal health.

Healthy lifestyle choices

Adopting a healthy lifestyle, which includes eating balanced food, staying hydrated, and avoiding harmful habits, benefits general health and resilience to stress-related issues.

Understanding the complex interaction between stress and renal health highlights the significance of overall well-being. Chronic stress, with its complicated physiological responses and potential kidney damage, emphasizes the importance of adopting stress management measures into daily life. Individuals can protect their renal health and improve their overall physical and mental well-being by proactively addressing stress through lifestyle changes, behavioral adjustments, and the adoption of good coping techniques. It is critical to consult with healthcare professionals for tailored guidance and assistance, especially if you have pre-existing renal disorders or are predisposed to stress-related health problems. Through these proactive strategies, individuals can manage the challenges of stress and promote long-term renal health.

Strategies for stress reduction

In today's fast-paced world, effective stress-reduction measures are critical to sustaining mental, emotional, and physical health. Chronic stress can have a significant impact on health, contributing to a variety of conditions ranging from cardiovascular disease to compromised immune function. This comprehensive discussion goes into a range of tactics that individuals can use to alleviate stress, increase resilience, and promote a balanced and harmonious life.

1. Mindfulness & Meditation

Mindful Awareness is the practice of paying attention to the current moment without passing judgment. Practices like mindful breathing and body scan meditation can help people manage stress by grounding them in the present moment.

Meditation Techniques: Studies have indicated that regular meditation, such as mindfulness meditation, loving-kindness meditation, and transcendental meditation, can help reduce stress and anxiety. These techniques encourage relaxation, focus, and inner peace.

2. Deep breathing exercises.

Diaphragmatic Breathing: Deep breathing exercises like diaphragmatic breathing (also known as belly breathing) help the body relax. This easy technique involves taking calm, deep breaths to promote relaxation and reduce the physiological impacts of stress.

Box breathing is a yoga and meditation practice that consists of inhaling, holding the breath, expelling, and holding the breath again—each for a count of four. This regular breathing pattern helps promote a sense of tranquility and equilibrium.

3. Regular physical activity.

Endorphin Release: Exercise is an effective stress-reduction technique. Physical activity causes the release of endorphins, which are the body's natural mood boosters. Regular movement, whether through cardiovascular exercise, weight training, or yoga, can help to reduce stress and enhance overall health.

Nature Walks and Outdoor Activities: Spending time in nature and participating in outdoor activities might help you get the benefits of exercise. Physical activity and exposure to the outdoors have been found to lower stress and improve mood.

4. Healthy Sleep Habits

Constant Sleep Schedule: Having a constant sleep schedule is essential for stress management. Adequate, quality sleep allows the body to heal and replenish, increasing resistance to stressors.

Creating a soothing Bedtime Routine: A soothing bedtime routine, which may include activities like reading, mild stretching, or practicing relaxation techniques, tells the body it's time to unwind.

5. Time Management:

Effective time management entails prioritizing tasks and focusing on the most important ones. This decreases feelings of overwhelm and allows people to more easily negotiate their everyday responsibilities.

Breaks and Downtime: Including breaks and downtime in everyday activities is critical. Short breaks during work or study sessions help avoid burnout and provide periods of relaxation, lowering stress levels.

6. Social Support and Connection.

Open Communication: Sharing feelings and experiences with trustworthy friends, family, or a mental health professional relieves stress. Open conversation promotes a sense of connection and understanding.

Socializing and forming supportive relationships are essential for emotional well-being. Positive social connections help to create a sense of belonging and lessen feelings of isolation.

7. Cognitive Behavioral Techniques.

Cognitive restructuring entails identifying and addressing problematic thought habits. Individuals can lessen stress by reframing negative thoughts.

Problem-Solving Skills: Learning good problem-solving techniques enables people to deal with stressors more proactively. Breaking down issues into manageable steps and exploring answers might help to alleviate emotions of helplessness.

8. Hobbies and Creative Outlets

Artistic Expression: Taking part in creative activities, such as art, music, writing, or other hobbies, allows you to express yourself and relax. Creative activities can be used as a therapeutic method of stress reduction.

Mindful Hobbies: Choosing hobbies that involve concentration and attention, such as gardening, cooking, or crafting, can be calming and help to reduce stress.

9. Relaxation techniques

Progressive Muscle Calm: This technique involves gradually tensing and then relaxing various muscle groups to promote both physical and mental calm.

Guided Imagery: This technique uses visualization to generate relaxing mental images. This approach aids individuals in creating a mental retreat, lowering stress and fostering a sense of calm.

10. Technology Detox

Regularly disconnecting from electronic devices, social media, and constant connectivity promotes mental health. Unplugging from technology can help you relax and practice mindfulness.

Establishing Boundaries: Limiting gadget usage, particularly before bedtime, promotes healthy sleep patterns and minimizes the stress associated with constant contact.

Incorporating a variety of stress-reduction tactics into daily living can improve overall well-being and resilience. It is critical to acknowledge that people respond differently to different tactics, thus a personalized approach is essential. Experimenting with various tactics and determining the ideal mix for an individual's specific needs can result in better stress management and a more balanced, fulfilling existence. Seeking expert help when necessary can help you establish a personalized stress-reduction strategy. Individuals can handle life's problems more easily and create a long-lasting sense of inner calm by prioritizing mental well-being and using proactive stress reduction methods.

CONCLUSION

Recap of key points

A Brief Overview of Renal Health

The kidneys are complex organs that are essential for maintaining homeostasis. They are made up of the renal cortex and the medulla. Regular urination, clear urine, and steady blood pressure are all signs of excellent kidney health.

Importance of Renal Diet.

A renal diet is essential for treating illnesses such as chronic kidney discase. To reduce renal stress, restrict your sodium, potassium, and phosphorus consumption. Prioritizing high-quality protein sources, such as lean meats, can help sustain renal function.

Overview of Renal Dietary Restrictions.

Maintaining sodium, potassium, and phosphorus levels is critical. It includes eating low-phosphorus fruits and vegetables, staying hydrated, and making informed decisions about whole grains and healthy fats.

Foods to Include on a Renal Diet

Incorporating high-quality proteins like fish and chicken, low-phosphorus fruits like berries, and whole grains promotes a healthy renal diet. Portion control and meal planning provide adequate nutrient intake.

Foods to limit or avoid.

Restricting high-sodium foods, regulating potassium and phosphorus consumption, and limiting processed and packaged foods are all necessary measures for renal diet limits.

Monitor and Adjust the Renal Diet

Regular check-ups with healthcare specialists offer individualized advice. Individual adjustments are done depending on health requirements and changes in renal function.

Smoothie Cleanser Guide

Introduction to Smoothie Cleansing: Kane's natural method of conquering chronic kidney illness with nutrition and smoothies might inspire and guide others seeking holistic renal health.

Benefits of Using Smoothies

Smoothies are nutritious and help you stay hydrated. They provide a handy and enjoyable way to add critical nutrients to the diet.

How Smoothies Can Improve Renal Health

Making smoothies with low potassium and phosphorus content, as well as nutrient-dense combinations, promotes kidney health. These recipes incorporate berries, apples, and cauliflower.

Smoothie Recipes for Renal Health.

A range of kidney-friendly smoothie recipes can be created by incorporating low-potassium foods like cucumber, blueberries, and watermelon, as well as low-phosphorus options like almond milk, kale, and pineapple.

Incorporating Smoothies into the Daily Routine

Enhancing daily nutrition and hydration with smoothies, ensuring balanced components, and making them a regular part of the routine all benefit kidney health.

Stress Reduction Strategies

Mindfulness and meditation approaches, such as loving-kindness meditation, can improve relaxation, focus, and inner calm.

Deep breathing exercises.

Incorporating diaphragmatic and box breathing as deep breathing exercises promotes relaxation and reduces the physiological consequences of stress.

Regular Physical Activity

Regular physical activity produces endorphins, which promote mental well-being. Combining exercise with outdoor activities improves stress reduction.

Healthy Sleeping Habits

Establishing consistent sleep cycles and nighttime habits improves overall well-being. Quality sleep helps the body heal and adapt to stress.

Effective Time Management

Prioritizing chores and implementing relaxation periods into daily routines might help prevent burnout and manage stress more effectively.

Social Support and Connections

Emotional well-being is heavily influenced by open communication and the development of supportive connections. Positive social connections decrease emotions of loneliness.

Cognitive Behavioral Techniques

Individuals who challenge negative beliefs and build problem-solving abilities are better able to manage stress.

Hobbies and Creative Outlets

Engaging in artistic expression and mindful hobbies allows relaxation, self-expression, and a therapeutic method of stress reduction.

Relaxation techniques

Using relaxation techniques such as progressive muscle relaxation and guided visualization increases both physical and mental relaxation.

Technology Detox

Taking regular breaks from electronic gadgets and setting limits on technology use aids in mental cleansing and stress reduction.

By incorporating a renal-friendly diet, embracing smoothie cleansers, and implementing effective stress reduction strategies, individuals can empower themselves on their health journey. The interaction of these components produces a synergistic impact, boosting kidney health while also encouraging resilience and a healthy mentality.

Encouragement for maintaining a renal-friendly lifestyle

Adopting a renal-friendly lifestyle is a transforming journey that goes beyond dietary limitations. It entails a comprehensive approach to total health and well-being. Encouragement is essential in maintaining this lifestyle, providing drive and support for people navigating the challenges of kidney health. In this final section, we discuss the importance of encouragement and how cultivating a positive mindset can help people on their renal-friendly journey.

Embracing a positive mindset: Understanding The Significance

Encouraging people to see a renal-friendly lifestyle as a positive investment in their health is critical. Rather than viewing it as a set of limitations, consider it a basis for a better, more vibrant life. Highlighting the long-term benefits can help to transform the narrative from one of limitation to empowerment.

Shifting perspectives

Encouragement requires an adjustment in viewpoint. Emphasizing the benefits of a renal-friendly lifestyle, such as increased energy, improved well-being, and the ability to halt the progression of kidney disease, helps people understand the value of their decisions. It turns the journey into an opportunity for good development.

Celebrating small victories.

Acknowledging Progress

Celebrating even the slightest accomplishments is critical for staying motivated. Whether it's following nutritional rules, increasing physical exercise, or successfully managing stress, every step forward deserves to be recognized. Acknowledging progress promotes a sense of accomplishment.

Building Confidence

Encouragement is essential for creating confidence. Celebrating little accomplishments gives people confidence in their ability to maintain a renal-friendly lifestyle. This positive reinforcement becomes a potent motivator for perseverance and resilience in the face of adversity.

Establishing Support Systems.

Family and friends.

When people share their journeys with supportive family and friends, they feel more encouraged. Creating a network that understands and values the struggles and triumphs makes the trip more doable. Friends and family members can provide emotional support and encouragement.

Healthcare professionals

Emphasizing the need for frequent check-ups and open contact with healthcare experts is critical. These professionals can provide individualized advice, track progress, and offer encouraging words based on particular health needs. Knowing they have a supported team of specialists provides a sense of security.

Creating a supportive environment

Creating a Renal-Friendly Home

Encouraging people to make their homes suitable for a renal-friendly lifestyle is empowering. From storing kidney-friendly foods to establishing a tranquil environment, the home transforms into a wellness haven. A supportive home environment fosters beneficial behaviors.

Joining Support Groups.

Promoting engagement in renal health support groups fosters a sense of community. Sharing your experiences, struggles, and accomplishments with others who understand the path creates a supportive environment. Support groups provide a forum for encouraging and sharing insights.

Educating and Empowering: Knowledge leads to empowerment.

Encouragement is directly related to knowledge. Empowering people to understand the reasoning behind renal-friendly suggestions enables them to make informed decisions. Providing educational resources and clarifying how each choice impacts kidney health lays the groundwork for long-term lifestyle adjustments.

Setting Realistic Goals.

Encouragement is most effective when individuals set attainable and realistic goals. Breaking down larger goals into smaller, more doable steps promotes a sense of accomplishment and supports the notion that a renal-friendly lifestyle is possible. Realistic goals help to keep motivation.

Developing Resilience in the Face of Challenges

Addressing Setbacks

Encouragement requires a proactive approach to setbacks and challenges. Understanding that occasional deviations from the renal-friendly plan may occur enables individuals to overcome setbacks and move forward. Fostering a mindset that sees failures as learning opportunities promotes growth.

Stress Management

Emphasizing the link between stress and kidney health promotes the use of stress-reduction techniques. Stress management becomes an essential component of the renal-friendly lifestyle, enhancing overall well-being. Encouraging the use of stress-relieving activities improves resilience.

Providing Ongoing Motivation

Personalized Encouragement

Encouragement is most successful when it is tailored to specific tastes and reasons. Finding what connects with each individual, whether through affirmations, visualizations, or personal achievements, is key to maintaining motivation. Personalized encouragement recognizes an individual's strengths and ambitions.

Regular check-ins

Encouragement includes regular self-reflection and check-ins. Individuals can monitor their progress, recognize accomplishments, and alter their goals as appropriate. This constant examination promotes accountability and offers possibilities for renewed motivation. Regular check-ins guarantee that the renal-friendly lifestyle stays dynamic and adaptable.

Encouragement is the foundation of living a renal-friendly lifestyle. Individuals may overcome the problems of food restrictions, stress management, and overall well-being by encouraging positive, applauding accomplishments, and providing continual support. The journey to kidney health is a marathon, not a sprint, and encouragement is the fuel that propels people ahead.

Understanding that a renal-friendly lifestyle is a constant journey rather than a destination allows people to embrace the process and appreciate the benefits to their kidney health. Individuals can build a mindset that not only preserves a renal-friendly lifestyle but also transforms it into a rewarding and powerful path toward long-term well-being, with the correct encouragement. Accepting encouragement as a constant companion on this journey enables people not only to maintain their kidney health but also to thrive in their whole sense of well-being and vitality.

Importance of consulting healthcare professionals for personalized advice.

Maintaining optimal health, especially when dealing with specific problems such as kidney health issues, necessitates a sophisticated and tailored approach. While general health information is useful, engaging with healthcare specialists for tailored advice becomes critical, particularly in the context of renal health and adherence to a renal diet. This final section delves into the multiple necessities of receiving help from healthcare specialists, concluding with underlining its relevance to the complexities of a renal diet.

1. Knowledge of Renal Health

Healthcare experts, particularly nephrologists and dietitians who specialize in renal health, provide a wealth of knowledge and expertise. Their in-depth expertise in renal function allows them to deliver individualized guidance based on individual health profiles and renal diseases.

2. Personalized Treatment Plans

One of the key advantages of talking with healthcare specialists is the creation of tailored treatment regimens. These plans are created after doing a complete examination of an individual's health, taking into account aspects such as age, pre-existing health issues, medications, and lifestyle. This personalized approach guarantees that interventions are appropriate for the patient's specific needs and health goals.

3. Monitor Disease Progression

Continuous monitoring is vital for people treating chronic illnesses like chronic kidney disease (CKD). Healthcare experts play an important role in monitoring illness progression, assessing the efficacy of treatment regimens, and making necessary modifications. This continual supervision is essential for improving outcomes and managing the changing character of renal health.

4. Medication Management.

Healthcare professionals manage drugs recommended for renal diseases. They monitor pharmaceutical efficacy, evaluate potential side effects, and make modifications as needed. This tailored oversight ensures that pharmaceuticals are both effective and safe for the individual, which improves overall health.

5. Nutritional guidance

Renal health frequently necessitates specialized dietary changes, and healthcare professionals, notably renal dietitians, provide detailed nutritional advice. This counsel, tailored to an individual's renal function, dietary preferences, and cultural factors, ensures that dietary modifications are not only beneficial but also long-term, making it an essential component of a renal diet.

6. Lifestyle recommendations

Beyond drugs and dietary changes, lifestyle variables have a substantial impact on renal health. Healthcare specialists can offer tailored advice on lifestyle changes, such as recommendations for physical activity, stress management, and sleep hygiene. These tailored lifestyle therapies improve general well-being and enhance the efficacy of a renal diet.

7. Prevention and Early Intervention.

Regular check-ups with healthcare specialists enable proactive steps to prevent the advancement of kidney problems or the onset of consequences. Early diagnosis of changes in health status permits prompt treatments, potentially reducing or mitigating possible problems before they worsen.

8. Emotional Support.

Managing chronic health issues frequently presents emotional challenges. Healthcare experts not only provide medical advice, but also emotional support and guidance. This holistic approach acknowledges the interdependence of mental and physical well-being, resulting in a more thorough and efficient healthcare experience.

9. Collaboration and Coordination.

Consulting healthcare experts encourages collaboration among the many specialists involved in a patient's care. This coordinated approach guarantees that all areas of health are evaluated and interventions are consistent. Regular communication among healthcare team members improves the quality and consistency of care, which is especially important when managing complicated disorders such as renal health.

10. Empowering Patients.

Empowerment is a critical component of individualized treatment. Healthcare workers inform patients about their medical issues, treatment alternatives, and lifestyle choices. This knowledge enables people to actively participate in their health management, make educated decisions, and change their lifestyles to support their overall well-being.

In the setting of a renal diet, empowerment becomes critical to long-term adherence and excellent health outcomes.

Renal Diet as a Personal Journey:

When considering the complexities of a renal diet, the significance of interacting with healthcare professionals for individualized recommendations becomes especially clear. A renal diet is not a one-size-fits-all approach; it must be tailored to individual health needs, dietary preferences, and cultural influences.

Healthcare providers play an important role in guiding people through this unique journey. From developing dietary regimens specific to renal function to offering ongoing support and monitoring, their knowledge ensures that people may efficiently negotiate the difficulties of a renal diet. Collaboration between healthcare professionals and individuals is a dynamic partnership that enables patients to take control of their health and make informed decisions that are tailored to their specific requirements.

To summarize, consultation with healthcare professionals is more than simply a step in managing renal health; it is the foundation of customized care and a critical component in the effective implementation of a renal diet. Healthcare experts' experience, guidance, and support considerably improve the overall well-being of those dealing with renal health issues, paving the way for a healthier and more satisfying life.